Practical
Hepato-Gastroenterology Prescriber

Practical
Hepato-Gastroenterology Prescriber

Mamun-Al-Mahtab
MBBS MSc MD FACG
Associate Professor
Department of Hepatology
Bangabandhu Sheikh Mujib Medical University
Dhaka, Bangladesh

Sheikh Mohammad Fazle Akbar
MBBS MD PhD
Principal Investigator
Department of Medical Sciences
Toshiba General Hospital
Tokyo, Japan

Foreword
Kamrul Hasan Khan

JAYPEE *The Health Sciences Publisher*

New Delhi | London | Philadelphia | Panama

Jaypee Brothers Medical Publishers (P) Ltd

Headquarters

Jaypee Brothers Medical Publishers (P) Ltd
4838/24, Ansari Road, Daryaganj
New Delhi 110 002, India
Phone: +91-11-43574357
Fax: +91-11-43574314
Email: jaypee@jaypeebrothers.com

Overseas Offices

J.P. Medical Ltd
83 Victoria Street, London
SW1H 0HW (UK)
Phone: +44-20 3170 8910
Fax: +44 (0) 20 3008 6180
Email: info@jpmedpub.com

Jaypee-Highlights Medical Publishers Inc
City of Knowledge, Bld. 235, 2nd Floor, Clayton
Panama City, Panama
Phone: +1 507-301-0496
Fax: +1 507-301-0499
Email: cservice@jphmedical.com

Jaypee Medical Inc
325 Chestnut Street
Suite 412, Philadelphia
PA 19106, USA
Phone: +1 267-519-9789
Email: support@jpmedus.com

Jaypee Brothers Medical Publishers (P) Ltd
17/1-B Babar Road, Block-B, Shaymali
Mohammadpur, Dhaka-1207
Bangladesh
Mobile: +08801912003485
Email: jaypeedhaka@gmail.com

Jaypee Brothers Medical Publishers (P) Ltd
Bhotahity, Kathmandu, Nepal
Phone: +977-9741283608
Email: kathmandu@jaypeebrothers.com

Website: www.jaypeebrothers.com
Website: www.jaypeedigital.com

Inquiries for bulk sales may be solicited at: jaypee@jaypeebrothers.com

Practical Hepato-Gastroenterology Prescriber
First Edition: **2017**
ISBN: 978-93-86150-70-7
Printed at Sanat Printers

To

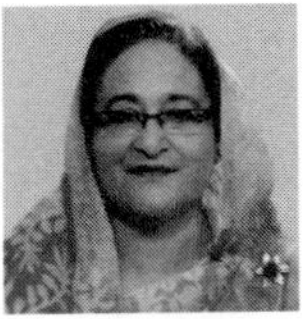 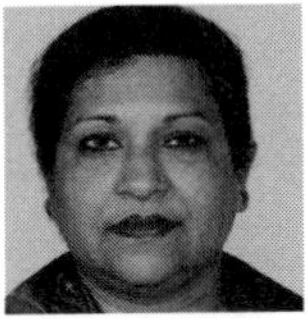

Sheikh Hasina *and* ***Sheikh Rehana***
the "light bearers" of
Bangabandhu's vision and wisdom.....

Contributors

Mohammad Abdur Rahim
MBBS MD (Hepatology)
Assistant Professor
Department of Hepatology
Abdul Malek Ukil Medical College
Noakhali, Bangladesh

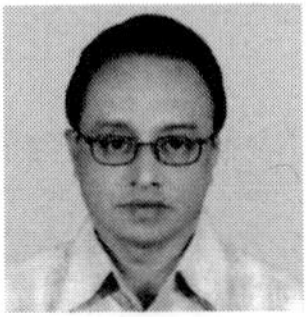

Sheikh Mohammad Noor-E-Alam
MBBS MD (Hepatology)
Assistant Professor
Department of Hepatology
Shaheed Tajuddin Ahmad Medical College
Gazipur, Bangladesh

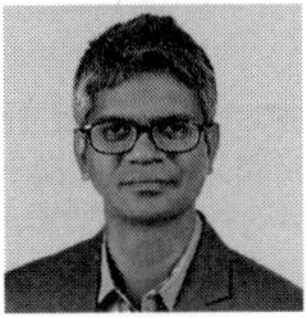

Mohammad Ashraful Alam
MBBS MD (Hepatology)
Assistant Professor
Department of Hepatology
Cox's Bazar Medical College
Cox's Bazar, Bangladesh

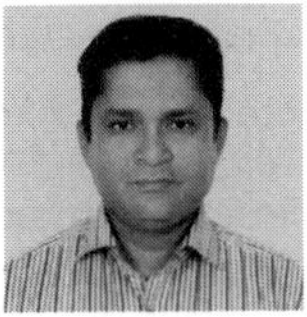

Faiz Ahmad Khondaker
MBBS MD (Hepatology) FCPS (Medicine)
Assistant Professor
Department of Hepatology
Shaheed Suhrawardy Medical College
Dhaka, Bangladesh

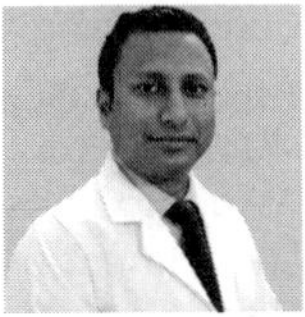

Ahmed Lutful Moben
MBBS MD (Hepatology)
Hepatologist
Kurmitola General Hospital
Dhaka, Bangladesh

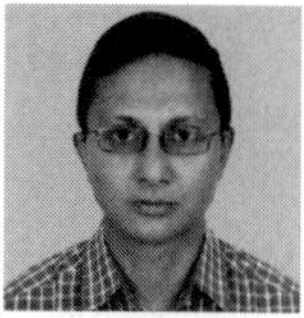

Ananta Shrestha
MBBS MD (Hepatology)
Consultant Hepatologist,
Alka Hospital
Kathmandu, Nepal

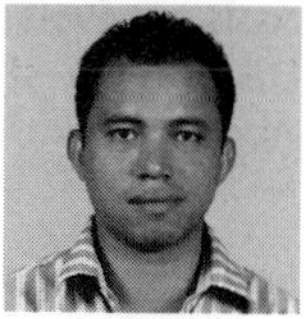

Mohammad Jahangir Alam Sarker
MBBS MD (Hepatology)
Assistant Professor
Department of Hepatology
Shaheed Suhrawardy Medical College
Dhaka, Bangladesh

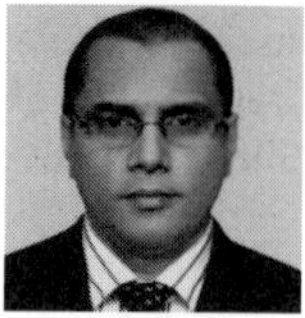

Mohammad Forhad Abedin
MBBS MD (Hepatology) FCPS (Medicine)
Resident Physician
Comilla Medical College
and Hospital
Comilla, Bangladesh

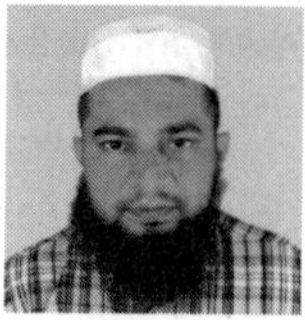

Utpal Das Gupta
MBBS MD (Hepatology) FCPS (Medicine)
Associate Consultant and Coordinator
Department of Gastroenterology and
Hepatology, Asgar Ali Hospital
Dhaka, Bangladesh

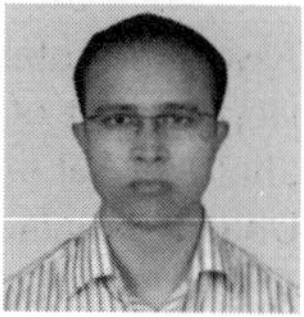

Thupten Kelsang Lama
MBBS MD (Hepatology)
Registrar
Department of Medicine (Hepatology Wing)
Civil Service Hospital, Minbhawan
Kathmandu, Nepal

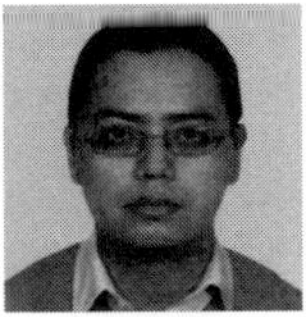

Mohammad Zia Hayder Bosunia
MBBS MD (Hepatology) FCPS (Medicine)
Assistant Professor,
Department of Hepatology
Rangpur Medical College
Rangpur, Bangladesh

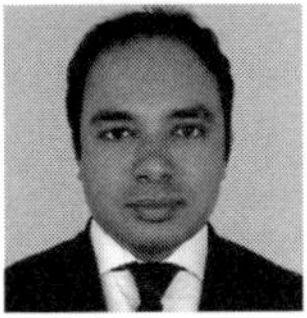

Abu Saleh Sadequl Islam
MBBS MD (Hepatology)
Assistant Professor
Department of Hepatology
SZR Medical College
Bogra, Bangladesh

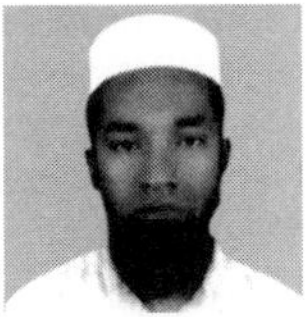

Syed Abul Foez
MBBS MD (Hepatology) FCPS (Medicine)
Assistant Professor
Department of Hepatology
Shaheed Syed Nazrul Islam Medical College
Kishoreganj, Bangladesh

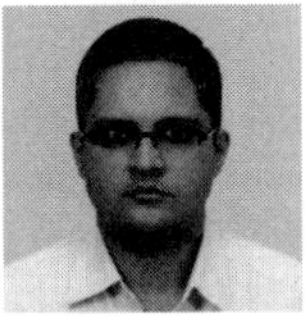

Foreword

The launch of a new book is always exciting. Although there are certain dominant leaders in the market, there are not too many ready reference books in hepatology and gastroenterology worldwide in relation to the enormous disease burden of these two specialties. I was, therefore, particularly pleased to be invited by a faculty member of my university and my direct students Dr Mamun-Al-Mahtab and Dr Sheikh Mohammad Fazle Akbar to write the foreword for a book conceived and brought into being by the enthusiasm and work of hepatologists from Bangladesh with contributions by a group of young postgraduates all of whom happen to be my students. The contents of this book shows an appreciation of the changing times in taking a global perspective of liver and gastrointestinal diseases as I am, my hope also is that the bringing together of the authorship of this book will help in fostering advancement of knowledge in hepatology and gastroenterology.

Kamrul Hasan Khan
Vice-Chancellor
Bangabandhu Sheikh Mujib Medical University
Dhaka, Bangladesh

Preface

Diseases of the liver and digestive system are common all over the world, more so in the developing countries, because of the extra burden of infections with diverse organisms. They present a challenge to the clinicians, who have a difficult task keeping themselves up-to-date with the progress.

Bearing this in mind, the task of preparing a ready reference book of diseases of the liver and digestive system, which can cater to the needs of all categories of doctors involved in the care of patients with diseases of these systems, has indeed become a necessity.

The book is intended for the specialists, postgraduate students and the general practitioners to update their knowledge. Our effort will be worthwhile if they find what they are looking for in this book.

Mamun-Al-Mahtab
Sheikh Mohammad Fazle Akbar

Contents

Section 5: Miscellaneous Disorders

Section 6: Diseases of Liver

Section 7: Diseases of Gallbladder and Biliary Tree

Section 8: Diseases of Pancreas

CHAPTER 1

Esophageal Candidiasis

- Generally present with dysphagia or odynophagia
- More common in immunocompromised patients, i.e. patients receiving chemotherapy, post-transplant antirejection medication and acquired immune deficiency syndrome (AIDS) patients
- *Candida albicans* is the most common cause
- Definitive diagnosis is established by upper gastrointestinal endoscopy, which reveals either focal or diffuse plaques in association with mucosal hyperemia and friability
- Biopsies show desquamated epithelial cells with typically appearing yeast forms; fungal invasion is usually present only in the superficial epithelium
- Treatment:
  - Oral fluconazole 100 to 200 mg/day for 14–21 days. Initially IV fluconazole can be given if unable to take orally. Alternatives for fluconazole-refractory disease includes itraconazole, voriconazole.

CHAPTER 2

Gastroesophageal Reflux Disease

- Heartburn: Retrosternal burning, commonly known as heart burn, and/or regurgitation after meal is the classical presentation
- Atypical manifestations: Asthma, chronic cough, chronic laryngitis, sore throat, and noncardiac chest pain
- Diagnostic tests are not needed with classical symptoms
- An empirical acid suppression trial is sufficient for diagnosis
- Upper GI endoscopy is needed with alarm symptoms, recurrent symptoms, atypical symptoms and high-risk for complications
- Complications: Barrett's metaplasia, esophageal stricture, esophageal adenocarcinoma
- Treatment:
  - Lifestyle modifications: Eating smaller meals and avoiding coffee, spicy and fatty foods, tomatoes, chocolate, alcohol, cigarettes
  - Avoid lying down within 3 hours after meals
  - Elevate head-end of bed on 6-inch blocks
  - Antacids and alginic acid
  - Oral H2-receptor antagonists
  - Once—daily oral proton pump inhibitor (PPI) taken 30 minutes before breakfast for 4–8 weeks
  - Symptoms relapse: Either continuous PPI, intermittent 2–4 week courses or on demand therapy.

Achalasia Cardia

- Motility disorder of esophagus
- Dysphagia starts slowly; worse on solids and eased by drinking liquids, standing and moving around after eating
- Episodes of chest pain due to esophageal spasm
- Nocturnal pulmonary aspiration
- Barium swallow shows tapered narrowing of the lower esophagus, dilated body; lower esophagus is aperistaltic and food filled
- Endoscopy indicated to exclude carcinoma of the cardia
- Treatment:
  - Endoscopic (forceful pneumatic dilatation, injection of botulinum toxin, peroral endoscopic myotomy)
  - Surgical (Heller's myotomy with partial fundoplication antireflux procedure
  - Proton pump inhibitor (PPI) therapy is necessary after surgery.

CHAPTER 4

Carcinoma Esophagus

- Sixth leading cause of death from cancers worldwide
- About 70% patients have extensive disease at presentation
- Two histologic types, squamous cell carcinoma and adenocarcinoma
- Highest-risk populations are in north central China, Iran and intervening central Asian countries
- Presents with dysphagia (90%), odynophagia (50%), anorexia, weight loss and cachexia
- Upper gastrointestinal (GIT) endoscopy and biopsy is the main tools for diagnosis
- Barium swallow X-ray can be done
- Primary therapy includes:
  - Surgery alone
  - Chemotherapy plus radiotherapy
  - Combined chemotherapy plus surgery or chemotherapy plus radiotherapy plus surgery
  - Endoscopic mucosal resection and/or PDT (stage 0, stage 1)
  - Palliative therapy includes:
    - Radiotherapy
    - Radiotherapy plus chemotherapy
    - Intraluminal brachytherapy
    - Endoscopic therapies.

CHAPTER 5

Peptic Ulcer Disease

- The male: female = 5:1 to 2:1 for duodenal ulcer and 2:1 or less for gastric ulcer
- Chronic gastric ulcer is usually single; 90% situated on the lesser curve within the antrum or at the junction between body and antral mucosa
- Chronic duodenal ulcer usually occurs in the first part of the duodenum and 50% are on the anterior wall
- Gastric and duodenal ulcers coexist in 10% patients and more than one peptic ulcer is found in 10–15% of patients
- Chronic condition with spontaneous relapses and remissions
- Recurrent abdominal pain with three notable characteristics, namely localization to epigastrium, relationship to food and episodic occurrence
- Anorexia and nausea, early satiety after meals or occasional vomiting especially in gastric outlet obstruction
- Endoscopy is preferred investigation and patients tested for *Helicobacter pylori* infection
- Breath tests or fecal antigen tests are best for accuracy, simplicity and noninvasiveness

- Treatment:
  - Cigarette smoking, aspirin and NSAIDs are to be avoided
  - *Helicobacter pylori* eradication— PPI taken simultaneously with two antibiotics (from amoxicillin, clarithromycin and metronidazole) for 10–14 days has success rate 80–90%
  - In rest 15–20%, a quadruple therapy regimen, consisting of omeprazole (or another PPI), bismuth subcitrate, metronidazole and tetracycline for 10–14 days
  - Third attempt is guided by antimicrobial sensitivity testing, rescue therapy (levofloxacin, PPI and clarithromycin) or long-term acid suppression
  - Surgical treatment:
    - Emergency (perforation, hemorrhage)
    - Elective (gastric outlet obstruction, persistent ulceration despite adequate medical therapy, recurrent ulcer following gastric surgery).

Zollinger-Ellison Syndrome

- Most common between 30 and 50 years of age and in both sexes
- Triad of severe peptic ulceration, gastric acid hypersecretion and non-β cell islet tumor of the pancreas (gastrinoma)
- One-half to two-thirds are malignant, but slow-growing
- Multiple endocrine neoplasia (MEN) type 1 present in 20–60% patients
- Severe and often multiple peptic ulcers in unusual sites
- Poor response to standard antiulcer therapy
- Bleeding and perforations are common
- Diarrhea is seen in one-thirdpatients
- Serum gastrin levels are grossly elevated (10–1000-fold)
- Injection of secretin causes paradoxical and dramatic increase in gastrin
- Tumor localization by endoscopic ultrasound (EUS) and radiolabeled somatostatin-receptor scintigraphy
- Treatment:
  - Small and single tumor can be resected
  - Continuous therapy with PPIs (double doses) can heal ulcers and alleviate diarrhea
  - Synthetic somatostatin analogue, octreotide by subcutaneous injection
  - Needs to be monitored for development of other manifestations of MEN 1.

CHAPTER 7

Gastritis/Gastropathy

- Nonsteroidal anti-inflammatory drug (NSAID), alcohol, medical or surgical illness and portal hypertension are the most common causes of erosive gastropathy
- Asymptomatic, may cause epigastric pain, nausea, vomiting, hematemesis or melena
- Upper gastrointestinal endoscopy shows thickened, edematous, nonpliable wall with erosions and reddened gastric folds
- Treatment:

  Stress gastritis
  - Patients with nasogastric tubes: Omeprazole (40 mg at 1 and 6 hours on day 1; then 40 mg once daily beginning on day 2)

  In hematemesis
  - Continuous infusions of a PPIs (esomeprazole or pantoprazole, 80 mg IV bolus, followed by 8 mg/h continuous infusion) as well as sucralfate suspension, 1 g orally every 4 to 6 hours

  NSAID gastritis
  - 2–4 weeks trial of an oral PPIs (omeprazole, rabeprazole, or esomeprazole 20–40 mg/day; lansoprazole 30 mg/day; pantoprazole, 40 mg/day)

Alcoholic gastritis

- H2-receptor antagonists, PPIsor sucralfate for 2–4 weeks

Portal hypertensive gastropathy (PHG)

- Propranolol, nadolo, or portal decompressive procedures.

CHAPTER 8

Functional Dyspepsia

- Chronic dyspepsia in the absence of organic disease
- Usually, young (<40 years), women:men = 2:1
- Nausea, early satiety, fullness, bloating after meals and no weight loss
- Morning symptoms are characteristic and occurs on waking
- There are no diagnostic points, apart perhaps from inappropriate tenderness on abdomen
- Patients often appear anxious. Pregnancy needs to be ruled out in young women
- All patients should be checked for *Helicobacter pylori* infection and patients >55 years should undergo endoscopy to exclude mucosal disease
- Ultrasound should be done to exclude gallstones
- Treatment:
  - 10% benefit from *H. pylori* eradication therapy
  - Metoclopramide (10 mg 3 times daily) or domperidone (10–20 mg 3 times daily), before meals if nausea, vomiting or bloating is prominent
  - H2-receptor antagonist if night pain or heartburn is troublesome
  - Low-dose tricyclic agents, such as amitriptyline may be helpful in up to two-thirds.

CHAPTER 9

Gastric Carcinoma

- Fourth leading cause of cancer death worldwide
- Incidence rises sharply after 50 years of age
- Risk factors include *H. pylori*, smoking, alcohol, nitrites, pernicious anemia, adenomatous gastric polyps, previous partial gastrectomy (>20 years), Ménétrier's disease,hereditary diffuse gastric cancer families (HDC-1 mutations), familial adenomatous polyposis
- Weight loss, weakness, ulcer-like pain, anorexia, nausea, early satiety, hematemesis, melena, dyspepsia, dysphagia, anemia are common
- Jaundice or ascites signifies metastatic spread
- Supraclavicular lymph nodes (Troisier's sign), umbilicus (Sister Joseph's nodule) or ovaries (Krukenberg tumor) may be present
- Paraneoplastic phenomena, such as acanthosis nigricans, thrombophlebitis (Trousseau's sign) and dermatomyositis can also be seen
- Metastases seen most commonly in liver, lungs, peritoneum and bone marrow.
- Upper gastrointestinal endoscopy: Diagnostic
- Computed tomography (CT): For intra-abdominal spread or

liver metastases

- Laparoscopy with peritoneal washings: For peritoneal spread
- Treatment:

  Surgery
  - Resection for early gastric cancers
  - Total gastrectomy with lymphadenectomy for locally advanced tumors
  - Distal esophagectomy for proximal tumors in the esophagogastric junction
  - Billroth I or Roux-en-Y reconstruction for small, distally located tumors

  Palliative treatment
  - Chemotherapy using 5-fluorouracil and cisplatin, ECF
  - Trastuzumab benefits patients whose tumors over-express human epidermal growth factor receptor-2 (HER2)
  - Endoscopic laser ablation to control dysphagia or recurrent bleeding
  - Carcinomas at the cardia and pylorus require endoscopic dilatation or expandable metallic stents
  - Nasogastric tube introduction for temporary relief of vomiting due to gastric outlet obstruction.

CHAPTER 10

Gastric Lymphoma

- Rare tumor, <5% of all gastric malignancies
- Common site for extranodal non-Hodgkin lymphoma
- 60% of all primary gastrointestinal lymphomas
- Lymphoid aggregates develop inpresence of *H. pylori* infection
- *H. pylori* infection is closely associated with development oflow-grade lymphoma (classified as extranodal marginal zone lymphomas of MALT type)
- Endoscopic ultrasound (EUS) isimportant in staging these lesions
- Clinical presentation is similar togastric cancer
- Endoscopically tumor appears as polypoid or ulcerating mass
- Treatment:
  - For low-grade lesions: *H. pylori* eradication and close observation; if (11:18) chromosomal translocations present, additional radiotherapy or chemotherapy
  - For high-grade B-cell lymphomas: Combination rituximab, chemotherapy, surgery and radiotherapy
  - Favorable prognosis in stage I and II disease, small resectable tumors, tumors with low-grade histology and age below 60 years.

CHAPTER 11

Celiac Disease

- T cell-mediated gluten intolerance in genetically susceptible individuals; may be associated with other HLA-linked autoimmune disease
- Clinical spectrum depends on extent and severity of small bowel involvement
- Some develop panmalabsorption, others develop nonspecific symptoms (e. g. oral ulceration, tiredness, weight loss, abdominal discomfort, diarrhea, excess flatulence)
- Children may present with delayed growth and puberty, malnutrition
- Gold standard for diagnosis: Mucosal biopsy of bulb, distal duodenum and proximal jejunum
- Serological tests: Anti-tissue transglutaminase IgA (anti-tTG), antiendomysial antibody IgA (anti-EMA)
- Complete blood count (CBC): Microcytic or macrocytic anemia, features of hyposplenism
- Biochemistry: Hypoalbuminemia, hypoprothrombinemia, hypocalcemia may be present

- Treatment:
  - Frequent dietary counseling to avoid wheat, barley, rye and oat gluten
  - Rice, corn, potatoes and soybeans are safe
  - Limit intake of dairy product until diarrhea disappears
  - Replace deficient micronutrients (e.g. folate, calcium, iron, vitamin-D)
  - Pneumococcal vaccination (if features of hyposplenism)
  - Repeat anti-tTG IgA and anti-EMA IgA after 12 months, usually disappear in compliant patient
  - In refractory case: Corticosteroids or immunosuppressive to induce remission.

CHAPTER 12

Small Intestinal Bacterial Overgrowth

- Defined as >10^5 CFU/mL of bacteria in the proximal small bowel
- Hypochlorhydria (long-term PPI use, partial gastrectomy, pernicious anemia), impaired motility (in diabetes, systemic sclerosis), surgical resection, fistule, hypogammaglobulinemia may predispose
- Presentation with diarrhea, steatorrhea, flatulence, weight loss and abdominal distension
- Quantitative culture of the duodenal fluid is the gold standard for diagnosis, but invasive and costly
- Noninvasively by hydrogen breath test
- Barium follow through or small bowel enema may reveal blind loop or fistulae
- Low serum vitamin B12 but normal or elevated folate level
- Treatment:
  - Surgical correction of fistulae or stricture
  - Antibiotics: Tetracycline (250 mg 4 times daily) or metronidazole (400 mg 3 times daily) or ciprofloxacin (250 mg twice daily) or rifaximine (400 mg 3 times daily) for 7 to 10 days; some require upto 4 weeks continuous rotating regimens

Patient with diabetes or scleroderma can benefit from anti-diarrheal (e.g. loperamide: 2 mg 4 to 6 times daily)

- In chronic case: IM vitamin B12 supplement
- Others: Probiotics, prokinetic agents.

Tropical Sprue

- Occuring in the tropics
- Small bowel bacterial overgrowth or alteration of intestinal flora may be responsible
- Presentations are non-specific and include diarrhea, steatorrhea, abdominal distension, anorexia, weight loss
- Remission and relapse are common
- In chronic cases, megaloblastic anemia, ankle edema, glossitis, stomatitis may be found
- No specific diagnostic test available
- Diagnosis relies on exclusion of celiac disease, endemic to the tropics where sanitation is suboptimal
- Treatment:
  - Combination of folic acid (5 mg/day) and tetracycline (250 mg 4 times daily for 28 days)
  - Correction of other nutritional deficiencies (vitamin B12, D and calcium)
  - Response to treatment usually prompt
  - In chronically ill patients, treatment should be prolonged (6 months to 1 year).

CHAPTER 14

Enteric Fever

- Enteric fever is produced by *Salmonella typhi* (typhoid fever) or occasionally by a serotype other than *S. typhi* (most often *S. paratyphi A, S. schottmuelleri,* or *S. hirschfeldii*)
- More common in Indian sub-continent, sub-Saharan Africa and Latin America
- Typhoid and paratyphoid fevers are transmitted by fecal-oral route
- Incubation period is 5 to 21 days (generally 7 to 14 days)
- Characterized by prolonged sustained fever (usually at 39.4° to 40° C (103° to 104° F or higher), relative bradycardia, splenomegaly, rose spots (30%) and leukopenia (20%)
- In the first week, usually there is fever, headache, myalgia, relative bradycardia, constipation, diarrhea and vomiting in children
- In the second week, there may be rose spots on trunk, splenomegaly, cough, abdominal distension, diarrhea
- After 2–3 weeks of illness, the severe complications of intestinal hemorrhage or perforation related to necrosis of Peyers patches may be observed in about 5% patients enteric fever
- Rarely complications may occur (e.g. pancreatitis, cholecystitis, infective endocarditis, pneumonia, hepatic or splenic abscess, orchitis, or focal infection at virtually any site)

- Diagnosis:
  - Best proved by isolation of the microorganism from blood (1st week), stool (3rd week) or bone marrow (95%)
  - The Widal (and other serologic) tests that detect serum antibodies against *S. typhi* are not very useful clinically as there is false-negative and false-positive results. Polymerase chain reaction (PCR) and other molecular techniques are not widely available.
- Treatment:
  - The fluoroquinolones (e.g. ciprofloxacin 500 mg twice daily or ofloxacin 400 mg orally twice daily) are the agents of choice for the treatment of enteric fever, but resistance is common, especially in the Indian sub-continent and also in UK
  - Third generation cephalosporins such as ceftriaxone (intravenously) are reliable alternatives
  - Alternative therapies that can be used are chloramphenicol, ampicillin, trimethoprim, sulfamethoxazole, and azithromycin
  - Patients often require supportive care with intravenous saline, correction of electrolyte and acid-base disturbances, and in the setting of intestinal bleeding, blood transfusion
  - If perforation is suspected, laparotomy should be performed as soon as possible to repair the perforation
  - Steroid therapy has shown to be beneficial in some patients with severe enteric fever and coma, delirium or shock
  - As steroids can mask the signs and symptoms of abdominal perforation these should not be continued for more than 48 hours.
- Prevention:
  - Improved sanitation and living conditions reduce incidence
  - Vaccination.

CHAPTER 15

Amebic Dysentery

- Most prevalent in tropical areas
- Most infections are asymptomatic
- Diarrhea begins gradually over one to several weeks, abdominal pain can occur even without diarrhea, fever is uncommon, weight loss is common
- There may be severe presentation with passage of blood and more extensive diarrhea
- Physical findings may reveal high fever, vomiting, abdominal pain, prostration, hepatomegaly, hypotension
- Microscopic examination of stool for identifying organism; identification of trophozoites or cysts in a symptomatic patient is highly suggestive
- Serologic assays are available with lower sensitivity (70%); cannot distinguish recent and old disease; Stool antigen test (Tech Lab II) has higher sensitivity (>90%)
- PCR-based tests are useful, but not generally available
- Colonoscopy may reveal typical flask-shaped ulcers with intact intervening friable mucosa; Fresh ulcer exudate should be examined for motile trophozoites and for *E. histolytica* antigen.

- Treatment:
  For asymptomatic intestinal infection
  - Luminal agent: Diloxanide furoate 500 mg orally three times daily for 10 days or iodoquinol 650 mg orally three times daily for 21 days or paromomycin,10 mg/kg orally three times daily for 7 days

  For mild to moderate intestinal infection
  - Metronidazole 750 mg orally three times daily or 500 mg intravenously every 6 hours for 10 days or tinidazole, 2 g orally daily for 3 days or nitazoxanide (useful alternative if the patient is intolerant to metronidazole or tinidazole) plus luminal agent

  Severe intestinal infection
  - Metronidazole 750 mg orally three times daily or 500 mg intravenously every 6 hours for 10 days or tinidazole, 1 g orally daily for 3 days plus luminal agent.

CHAPTER 16

Bacillary Dysentery

- Caused by *Shigellae*—Gram-negative rods
- Four groups: *Shigellae dysenteriae, flexneri, boydii* and *sonnei*
- Low infecting dose of around 10 organisms
- Spread may occur *via* contaminated food or flies, but transmission by unwashed hands after defecation is by far the most important factor
- Clinical features: Disease severity varies from mild to severe; presents with bloody diarrhea, fever, colicky abdominal pain and tenesmus
- Treatment:
  - Oral rehydration therapy or, if necessary, intravenous water and electrolyte replacement
  - Ciprofloxacin 500 mg twice daily orally for 3 days
  - Antidiarrheal medication should be avoided
  - Proper handwashing is important to prevent disease.

CHAPTER 17

Cholera

- Toxin-mediated acute watery diarrhea produced by *Vibrio cholerae* serotype O1
- Spreads *via* stool or vomit of symptomatic patients or subclinical cases
- Transmitted by infected drinking water, shellfish and food
- Severe diarrhea without pain or colic, vomiting; typical 'rice water' material is passed; may lead to severe dehydration, shock and oliguria
- 'Cholera sicca' occurs, with loss of fluid into dilated bowel, without typical gastrointestinal symptoms
- Dark-field microscopy of stool shows typical 'shooting star' motility of *V. cholerae*
- Rectal swab or stool cultures allow identification
- Treatment:
  - Replacement of water and electrolytes; Ringer-lactate is the best fluid
  - Vomiting usually stops once the patient is rehydrated
  - Total fluid requirements may exceed 50 L over a period of 2–5 days; 'Cholera cot' can facilitate accurate record
  - Antibiotic: Tetracycline 250 mg 4 times daily for three days ciprofloxacin 1 gm

- Prevention:
  - Strict personal hygiene and safe drinking water is vital
  - Flies must be denied access to food
  - Vaccination with a killed suspension of *Vibrio cholerae*.

Traveler's Diarrhea

- Travelers' diarrhea, affects people (20–50%) traveling outside their own countries, particularly to developing countries
- Infection is usually food or water-borne and younger travelers are often affected
- Disease usually lasts for 2–5 days, benign and self-limiting
- Onset is sudden with abdominal cramps, anorexia and watery diarrhea
- Defined as the passage of three or more unformed stools per day in a resident of an industrialized country traveling in a developing nation
- Most common cause is enterotoxigenic *Escherichia coli* (ETEC); other causes are *Shigella* species, *Salmonella* species, *Campylobacter* species, and viral pathogens
- Treatment:
  - Quinolone antibiotics may hasten recovery, but is not normally necessary
  - Rifaximin can also be used
  - Oral or IV rehydration fluid, if needed.
- Prophylaxis:
  - Prophylactic antibiotic therapy may also be effective for short stays, but should not be used routinely

Bismuth subsalicylate is an inexpensive agent for the prophylaxis of traveler's diarrhea [2 prophylaxis tablets (525 mg) four times a day].

- Prevention:
  - Improvements in hygiene
  - Eating only hot, freshly cooked food
  - Avoiding raw vegetables, salads and unpeeled fruits
  - Drinking only boiled or treated water and avoiding ice.

CHAPTER 19

Abdominal Tuberculosis

- Although any portion of the gastrointestinal tract may be affected, terminal ileum and cecum are the sites most commonly involved
- Active pulmonary disease is present in <50% of patients
- Patients may be without symptoms or complain of acute or chronic abdominal pain and swelling, obstructive symptoms, hematochezia, weight loss and diarrhea
- A palpable mass in the abdomen is a common finding at presentation
- Nonspecific abdominal pain, fever, and ascites should raise the suspicion of tuberculous peritonitis
- Granulomatous hepatitis occurs occasionally
- Intestinal tuberculosis may cause mucosal ulcerations or scarring and fibrosis with narrowing of the lumen
- Complications include intestinal obstruction, hemorrhage and perianal disease with fistula. A 'doughy abdomen' due to extensive intra-abdominal inflammation may also be detected
- Barium radiography (better for hyperplastic type) may demonstrate mucosal ulcerations, thickening or stricture formation
- Abdominal CT may show thickening of the cecum and ileocecal valve and massive lymphadenopathy and elevated ESR

- Raised SGPT suggests hepatic involvement
- Colonoscopy (better for ulcerated type) may demonstrate an ulcerated mass, multiple ulcers with steep edges and adjacent small sessile polyps, small ulcers or erosions, or small diverticula, most commonly in the ileocecal region
- Diagnosis is established by either endoscopic or surgical biopsy revealing acid-fast bacilli, caseating granuloma, or positive cultures from the organism
- Detection of tubercle bacilli in biopsy specimens by PCR is now the most sensitive means of diagnosis
- Gene Xpert test can be done from peritoneal fluid
- Treatment with standard antituberculous regimens is effective
- There is no obvious role of steroids; in both types chemotherapy is the curative, but when there are features of obstruction or perforation, then operative treatment is required.

CHAPTER 20

Radiation Enteritis

- Can occur with radiation treatment of rectal, cervical, uterine, prostate, urinary bladder and testicular cancers
- Relatively immobile rectosigmoid colon is highly susceptible to radiation injury
- Risk depends on total dose, dosing schedule and concomitant chemotherapy
- Acute injury typically occurs within 6 weeks and is manifested by diarrhea, tenesmus and rarely bleeding
- Chronic radiation proctopathy can occur nearly a year following therapy and associated with rectal pain, bleeding, diarrhea and obstructed defecation
- Barium follow through: Used to diagnose fistulae, small bowel strictures and ulcer
- In acute phase, rectal changes and extent of lesion can be assessed by sigmoidoscopy/colonoscopy
- Treatment:
  - In acute phase: Oral and topical sucralfate, oral and topical steroids, 5-ASA, sulfasalazine, hyperbaric oxygen and antibiotics (metronidazole)
  - For bleeding: Argon laser photocoagulation, heater probe, bipolar cautery and formaldehyde application

- Diarrhea can be managed by loperamide or codeine phosphate
- Stool softeners can be used in patients with obstructive symptoms
- Others: Blood transfusion, oral iron, nutritional supplement
- Surgery: Indicated in case of obstruction, perforation and fistula.

CHAPTER 21

Crohn's Disease

- Segmental granulomatous inflammation affecting any part of the GI tract, special predisposition for the terminal ileum, colon and ano-rectum with patchy distribution (skip lesions)
- Presentation generally includes: Abdominal pain and tenderness (classically right lower quadrant), intermittent non-bloody diarrhea, weight loss, anemia, glossitis, angular stomatitis, abdominal mass
- Inflammation is through all layers of bowel wall and may result in fissure, fistulae, abscess
- May have extraintestinal manifestations: Sacroilitis, peripheral arthritis, episcleritis, uveitis, erythema nodosum, pyoderma gangrenosum, sclerosing cholangitis, mouth ulcer
- Colonoscopy with biopsy remains mainstay to confirm diagnosis and define disease extent
- Abdominal plain X-ray films are useful for detecting obstruction and megacolon
- Small bowel barium series are useful for imaging strictures, fistulae
- CT abdomen and pelvis allows imaging the bowel wall as well as extraluminal mass and abscess
- There may be anemia, leukocytosis, thrombocytosis, raised erythrocyte sedimentation rate (ESR), C-reactive protein (CRP), low albumin

- Fecal lactoferrin and calprotectin are promising markers to distinguish from IBS and for monitoring therapy
- Treatment:

  For inducing clinical remission
  - Prednisolone: 40–60 mg/day, after 2 weeks tapered by 5 mg/week

  In case of severe disease
  - Intravenous methylprednisolone (40–60 mg/day) or hydrocortisone (200–300 mg/day) or IV infliximab (5 mg/kg at 0, 2 and 6 weeks with 8 weekly maintenance thereafter)

  Maintenance therapy
  - Azathioprine (2–2.5 mg/kg/day) or 6 mercaptopurine (1–1.5 mg/kg/day) or methotrexate (IM/SC 15–25 mg/week)
  - Stop smoking

  For simple perianal disease
  - Ciprofloxacin (500 mg twice daily) and/or metronidazole (1–1.5 g/day)

  Abscess, fistulae, perforation and obstruction
  - Surgery is indicated.

CHAPTER 22

Ulcerative Colitis

- Inflammatory disorder involving mucosal layers of the colon
- From the rectum inflammation extending proximally in a confluent manner
- Frequently acute or subacute in onset followed by relapse and remission
- Clinical features: Depends on extent and severity of involvement; overt rectal bleeding and tenesmus are universal, mild abdominal tenderness (usually in the hypogastrium and left lower quadrant); digital rectal examination shows visible red blood; severe abdominal pain, tenderness, fever, tachycardia suggest fulminant colitis or toxic megacolon
- May have extraintestinal manifestation like Crohn's disease
- Abdominal plain X-ray films are useful in fulminant colitis (thumb-printing)
- Flexible sigmoidoscopy/colonoscopy allows assessment of the extent and severity; dysplastic or frankly malignant polyps/mass also found frequently
- Treatment:

  Fulminant colitis

  - Hospitalization, monitor jointly by physician and surgeon

- Intravenous fluid, nutritional support, correction of anemia and electrolytes imbalance, antibiotics, subcutaneous low-molecular-weight heparin
- Start IV corticosteroids (methylprednisolone 60 mg or hydrocortisone 400 mg daily; if not responding within 3–5 days consider infliximab (5 mg/kg) or cyclosporine (2 mg/kg)
- Urgent colectomy: if no response after 7–10 days.

Mild to moderately active disease

- Oral and topical 5-aminosalicylic acid (5-ASA) (top and tail approach); if no response within 2–4 weeks oral prednisolone (40 mg/day, tapered by 5 mg/week)

Maintenance of remission

- Oral 5-ASA is preferred first line agent
- If frequent relapse, consider thiopurines (6-MP or azathioprine)

Surgery

- Total proctocolectomy indicated in refractory cases and if associated with dysplasia or malignancy.

CHAPTER 23

Diverticulosis

- Middle-aged people are mostly affected
- Sigmoid and descending colon are common sites
- May be asymptomatic; complicated diverticulosis like acute diverticulitis, pericolic abscess, bleeding, perforation or stricture are uncommon
- Refined diet without fiber is responsible for the condition
- Diverticula consist of protrusions of mucosa covered by peritoneum
- Impaction of diverticula with fecoliths cause inflammation
- Clinical features: Constipation with colicky pain in suprapubic region or left iliac fossa, palpable sigmoid colon, tenderness, guarding, rigidity or palpable mass in left side; sometimes there is diarrhea, rectal bleeding or fever
- Differential diagnosis: Colorectal cancer, ischemic colitis, inflammatory bowel disease (IBD) and infection
- Complication: Perforation, pericolic abscess, fistula formation or acute rectal bleeding
- Investigations: Barium enema to confirm the presence of diverticula, strictures and fistulae; flexible colonoscopy is necessary to exclude coexisting neoplasm
- In severe diverticulosis, colonoscopy requires expertise and carries risk of perforation

- Computed tomography is used to assess complications such as perforation or pericolic abscess
- Treatment:
  - Asymptomatic disease requires no treatment
  - High-fiber diet, ispaghula husk, 1–2 sachets daily taken with plenty of fluids
  - Antispasmodics to relieve spasm
  - Acute attacks of diverticulitis should be treated with 7 days of metronidazole (400 mg 3 times daily orally), along with co-amoxiclav (500/125 mg 4 times daily)
  - Intravenous fluids, intravenous antibiotics, analgesia and nasogastric suction for severe cases
  - Emergency surgery may be needed for severe hemorrhage or perforation
  - Acute paracolic abscesses may need percutaneous drainage
  - Elective surgery may be done for repeated attacks of obstruction once the acute episode has settled.

CHAPTER 24

Appendicitis

- Peak incidence in the 2nd and 3rd decades of life
- Result from appendiceal luminal obstruction, most commonly caused by a fecalith
- Vague or colicky periumbilical or epigastric pain shifts to the right lower quadrant within 12 hours
- Nausea, vomiting, low-grade fever; localized tenderness in the right-lower quadrant; the 'psoas sign' (pain on passive extension of the right hip) and the 'obturator sign' (pain with passive flexion and internal rotation of the right hip) are strongly suggestive of appendicitis
- Atypical presentation in retrocecal appendicitis, pelvic appendicitis, in elderly patients and in pregnancy
- Moderate leukocytosis with neutrophilia; microscopic hematuria and pyuria are present in 25% of patients
- Both abdominal ultrasound and CT scanning are useful for diagnosis
- Gastroenteritis, acute salpingitis or tubo-ovarian abscess, twisted ovarian cyst, ruptured ectopic pregnancy, ureteral colic or pyelonephritis, diverticulitis, Meckel diverticulitis, carcinoid of the appendix, perforated colonic cancer, Crohn's ileitis, perforated peptic ulcer, cholecystitis, and mesenteric adenitis are usual differential diagnosis

Treatment.
- Uncomplicated appendicitis: Appendectomy is the mainstay of treatment; laparoscopic appendicectomy is preferred
- Prior to surgery, should give broad-spectrum antibiotics with Gram-negative and anerobic coverage
- Recommended preoperative intravenous regimens include cefoxitin 1–2 g every 8 hours; ampicillin-sulfbactam 3 g every 6 hours; or ertapenem 1 g as a single dose
- Emergency appendectomy for perforated appendicitis with generalized peritonitis
- Interval appendectomy after 6 weeks to prevent recurrent appendicitis.

• Prognosis: Mortality rate from uncomplicated appendicitis is extremely low; even in perforated appendicitis, mortality rate is low except in the elderly where it may be upto 15%.

CHAPTER 25

Rectal Polyp

- May be nonneoplastic or neoplastic (<1%)
- Divided into 3 groups: Hyperplastic polyps, adenomas and polyposis syndromes
- Hyperplastic polyps posses some malignant potential in the setting of hyperplastic polyposis syndrome
- Adenomas comprise about 10% of polyps; small polyps have small potential, but larger polyps have more potential of having cancer
- Adenomas are traditionally divided histologically into 3 types—tubular, tubulovillous, and villous
- Villous adenomas tend to be larger and associated with the highest morbidity and mortality; can cause hypersecretory syndromes with hypokalemia
- Polyps >1 cm contain substantial villous component or have high grade dysplasia and carry increased risk of cancer
- Polyposis syndromes are hereditary conditions that include familial adenomatous polyposis (FAP), hereditary nonpolyposis colorectal cancer (HNPCC)/Lynch syndrome, Gardner syndrome, Turcot syndrome, Peutz-Jeghers syndrome, Cowden disease, familial juvenile polyposis and hyperplastic polyposis
- Some genetic factors contribute to the development of these syndromes

- Risk for malignant progression is much greater with multiple polyps compared to the risk with isolated colonic polyps
- Signs and symptoms:
  - Most patients are asymptomatic
  - Rectal bleeding may be associated with iron deficiency anemia
  - Diarrhea or constipation
  - Distal rectal polyps may be detected by digital rectal examination.
- Diagnosis:
  - Stool occult blood test
  - Flexible sigmoidoscopy: Good screening test
  - Colonoscopy: Preferred test to detect colonic polyps, obtain biopsies and/or perform endoscopic resection
  - Capsule endoscopy
  - Stool DNA
- Management:
  - Polypectomy: For solitary pedunculated polyp
  - Colonic resection: Multiple intestinal polyps associated with Familial adenomatous polyposis (FAP)
- Mortality/Morbidity:
  - Untreated, colonic polyps can progress to carcinoma over several years
  - Morbidity: Bleedings, diarrhea, intestinal obstruction
- Surveillance:
  - Surveillance colonoscopy should be undertaken at 3–5-year intervals
  - Once all polyps have been removed, surveillance colonoscopy should be undertaken at 3–5-year intervals.

CHAPTER 26

Colorectal Cancer

- Common type of internal malignancy
- Common over the age of 50 years
- Multifactorial disease process. Environmental (including, diet) and genetic factors are important
- Clinical features:
  - Fresh rectal bleeding, anemia from occult bleeding, altered bowel habit, mucus discharge or a feeling of incomplete rectal emptying, colicky lower abdominal pain, intestinal obstruction or perforation
  - Physical examination may reveal anemia and/or weight loss, palpable abdominal mass, hepatomegaly, ascities from metastases. Low rectal tumors may be palpable on digital examination.
- Investigations:
  - Investigation of choice is colonoscopy with biopsy of suspicious lesions
  - CT colonography (virtual colonoscopy) for patients in whom colonoscopy is incomplete and those who are at high-risk of complications
  - CT of chest, abdomen and pelvis, endoanal ultrasound, positron emission tomography (PET) including PET-CT fusion scan for staging

- Carcinoembryonic antigen (CEA) levels are of limited value in diagnosis, but helpful during follow-up

- Modified Dukes classification:

Dukes stage	***A***	***B***	***C***	***D***
Definition	Tumor confined within bowel wall	Extension through bowel wall	Tumor involving lymph nodes	Distant metastases
5-year survival rate (%)	>90	65	30–35	<5

- Management:
  - Surgery is the curative treatment for localized colon cancer
  - Neoadjuvant radiotherapy or chemoradiotherapy for locally advanced rectal cancer
  - Metastatic disease confined to liver or lung should be considered for resection
  - Postoperative colonoscopy after 6–12 months and then at 5 years to search for local recurrence or development of new lesions.
- Palliation of advanced disease:
  - Palliative surgery of the primary tumor even with metastases may need to treat obstruction, bleeding or pain
  - Palliative chemotherapy with 5-fluorouracil/folinic acid, capecitabine, oxaliplatin or irinotecan improves survival
  - Monoclonal antibodies using bevacizumab or cetuximab, either alone or together with chemotherapy for advanced metastatic disease

  - Pelvic radiotherapy for distressing rectal symptoms such as pain, bleeding or severe tenesmus
  - Endoscopic laser therapy or expandable metal stent can be used to relieve obstruction
- Prevention and screening:
  - Secondary prevention aims to detect and remove lesions at an early or premalignant stage
  - Several potential methods exist:
    - Population-based screening of people over the age of 50 years by regular fecal occult blood (FOB) testing
    - Colonoscopy remains the gold standard
    - Flexible sigmoidoscopy is an alternative option
    - Screening for high-risk patients by molecular genetic analysis.

Anal Fissure

- An anal fissure is a tear or ulcer in the lining of the anus
- Located commonly in midline, posteriorly (90%)
- Constipation, muscle spasm, anal sex are usual causes
- Fissures cause pain and bleeding, usually during or shortly after bowel movement
- Pain lasts for several minutes to several hours and then subsides until the next bowel movement
- Diagnosed by gentle inspection of anus
- Treatment:
  - May not be needed
  - Stool softeners
  - Applying topical anesthesia to anus after defecation
  - Applying nitroglycerin ointment to the area of fissure
  - Injection botulinum toxin may be used to reduce sphincter spasm
  - If above measures fail, surgery may be needed.

CHAPTER 28

Hemorrhoids

- Dilated veins occurring in relation to the anus
- Internal or external
- Internal hemorrhoids: Bright red painless bleeding, principal and earliest symptoms
  - 1st degree: Bleed, but do not prolapse
  - 2nd degree: Prolapse on defecation, but return or have to be replaced manually and stay reduced
  - 3rd degree: Prolapsed permanently
  - Mucoid discharge, pruritus, pain (if complications supervene), anemia rarely.
- External hemorrhoids: Visible at the anal verge, usually no symptoms, may be associated with acute pain and new lump from thrombosis
- Symptomatic hemorrhoids may appear during pregnancy, in carcinoma rectum, from chronic constipation and straining at micturition
- Treatment:
  - Dietary manipulation: High fiber diet along with 6–8 glasses of non-alcoholic, non-caffined fluid daily
  - Avoid excessive straining and reading during defecation
  - Avoid medications that promote bleeding (e.g. NSAIDs)
  - Flavonoids (Diosmin and hesperidin): Questionable benefit, used for relief of acute symptoms

- If fails, aggressive non-surgical treatment: Sclerotherapy, rubber-band ligation, cryotherapy, infrared photocoagulation
- Surgical treatment: 3rd degree internal hemorrhoids
- Thrombosed external hemorrhoids: Sitz bath, analgesics, topical application of 0.3% nifedipine cream
- If fails, surgery.

CHAPTER 29

Aphthous Ulcer

- Superficial, painful and recurrent ulcers
- Occur anywhere inside the mouth
- Treatment:
  - No treatment may be needed
  - Avoid spicy foods, citrous fruit drinks and very salty foods
  - Chlorhexidine mouthwash twice a day
  - Steroid lozenge
  - Topical corticosteroids (0.1% triamcinolone in orabase)
  - Choline salicylate 8.7% gel
  - Oral corticosteroids.

Nausea and Vomiting

- Common causes: Gastroduodenal (peptic ulcer disease, gastric cancer, gastroparesis), acute abdomen (appendicitis, cholecystitis, pancreatitis), uremia, infections (hepatitis, gastroenteritis, urinary tract infection), drugs (NSAIDs, opiates, digoxin, antibiotics, cytotoxins), CNS disorders (vestibular neuronitis, migraine, raised intracranial pressure, meningitis), Metabolic (diabetic ketoacidosis, Addison's disease, cyclical vomiting syndrome), alcoholism, psychogenic
- Treatment:
  - Hospitalization for severe dehydration, if oral fluid replenishment cannot be sustained
  - If oral intake is tolerated, oral feeding started with liquids with low fat content
  - Motion sickness, inner ear disease: Dimenhydrinate, meclizine
  - Medication, toxin or metabolic-induced emesis: Prochlorperazine, thiethylperazine
  - Chemotherapy-induced nausea and vomiting: Ondansetron, granisetron, lorazepam, methylprednisolone, dexamethasone, tetrahydrocannabinol
  - Chronic idiopathic nausea, cyclic vomiting syndrome: Amitriptyline, nortriptyline
  - Gastroparesis: Metoclopramide, erythromycin, domperidone, mirtazapine.

CHAPTER 31

Hiccup

- Due to involuntary contraction of the diaphragm several times per minute, also known as chronic synchronous diaphragmatic flutter (SDF)
- Clinical features: May present as single or series of breathing diaphragmatic spasms of varying spacing and duration or brief, unexpected, shoulder, abdomen, throat or whole body tremor. May also present as audible hupp or as brief but distracting or painful, occasional disruption of breathing
- Causes: Coughing, rapid eating, intense emotion, carbonated beverage, laughing, etc. Systemic causes are chronic cough, kidney failure, stroke, liver failure, multiple sclerosis, meningitis, gastroesophageal reflux disease (GERD)
- Treatment: Usually treated at home through self-care; medically treated in severe and persistent cases; useful drugs are metoclopramide, gabapentin, proton pump inhibitors; haloperidol, metoclopramide, and chlorpromazine are effective in intractable hiccup; persistent rectal digital message and intranasal vinegar effective for chronic and severe hiccup; treatment of cause underlying disease is needed.

Irritable Bowel Syndrome

- Recurrent abdominal discomfort or pain
- Improvement of pain with defecation
- Patient experience diarrhea or constipation or mixed type symptoms
- Patients may complain of bloating, belching, flatus, abdominal distention, mucus per rectum, feeling of incomplete emptying
- Absence of alrming features like nocturnal symptoms, rectal bleeding, dysphagia, recurrent vomiting, weight loss, family history of colon cancer
- Physical findings that virtually excludes irritable bowel syndrome (IBS) are presence of anemia, abdominal mass, active arthritis, thyroid dysfunction
- Treatment:
  - Provide a positive diagnosis to patient; reassure and explain nature of illness to patient
  - Avoid excess fatty foods, caffeine or alcohol
  - For diarrhea predominant IBS: Antidiarrheal drugs like tablet loperamide 2–16 mg/day or cholestyramine 1 sachet/day, tablet codeine phosphate 30–90 mg/day, tablet Rifaximin 400–600 mg daily for 10 to 14 days, if symptoms persist

  - For constipation predominant IBS: Fiber supplement, e.g. Ispaghula (psyllium hydrophilic mucilloid), polyethylene glycol, tab lubiprostone 8 µgm twice daily.
  - For pain: Mebeverine or dicyclomine or propantheline or hyoscyamine
  - Pippermint oil, antidepressant and anxiolytics (tablet amitryptyline or imipramine or nortryptyline; starting dose 10–25 mg, increase dose 10–25 mg weekly or tablet duloxetine 30–60 mg at night)
  - Psycological therapy.
- Probiotics have some role.

CHAPTER 33

Constipation

- Infrequent bowel movement (≤3 times/week) or passing of stool less than the person's normal habit or with difficulty, with straining or pain
- History of drugs, dietary habits, diabetes, chronic laxative use, anxiety/depression, symptoms suggestive of hypothyroidism must be evaluated
- Indications for investigation: Age >40 years, change in bowel habit, associated symptoms (weight loss, per-rectal mucus or blood, tenesmus)
- For every patient direct rectal examination (DRE) must be carried out (in case of obstruction rectum may be completely empty; while with functional constipation, rectum may contain hard rock fecal mass)
- Constipation unlikely to be the sole symptom of serious disease if digital rectal exam (DRE), erythrocyte sedmentation rate (ESR) and serum TSH are normal
- Treatment:
  - Reassurance
  - Lifestyle modification: Increased dietary fiber, exercise, fluid intake, encouraging dedicated bathroom time

- For chronic constipation: Laxatives, stool softners, suppositories (e.g. glycerine), probiotics, lubiprostone
- Surgery: In highly selected patient (e.g. Hirschsprung disease, pelvic floor inertia)
- Treatment of the primary cause (e.g. hypothyroidism, diabetes).

CHAPTER 34

Hepatocellular Jaundice

- Common causes:
  - Viral infections: Hepatitis A, B ± D, C and E, cytomegalovirus (CMV), Epstein-Barr virus (EBV), herpes simplex, yellow fever
  - Drugs: Paracetamol, halothane, antituberculous drugs, ecstasy, herbal
  - Poisons: *Amanita phalloides*
  - Miscellaneous: Wilson's disease, acute fatty liver of pregnancy, shock and cardiac failure, Budd-Chiari syndrome, leptospirosis, lymphoma
  - Cryptogenic
- Diagnosis of viral hepatitis:
  - Nonspecific prodromal symptoms, like headache, myalgia, arthralgia, nausea, vomiting and diarrhea
  - Abdominal discomfort, dark urine, pale stools
  - Tender hepatomegaly, occasionally mild splenomegaly
  - Hepatitis E during pregnancy is associated with active liver failure (ALF) and has high mortality
  - Complications: ALF, cholestasic hepatitis (hepatitis A), aplastic anemia, chronic liver disease and cirrhosis (hepatitis B and C), relapsing hepatitis

- Abnormal LFTs and viral markers like anti-HAV IgM, HBsAg, anti-HBc IgM, HBV DNA, anti-HCV, anti-HEV IgM and USG.
- Treatment of acute viral hepatitis:
  - Most individuals do not need hospital care
  - Sedatives and narcotics should be avoided
  - No specific dietary modification needed
  - Patients with severe nausea or vomiting must be hydrated with IV fluid
  - Alcohol should be avoided during acute illness
    - Elective
  - Surgery should be avoided in case of acute viral hepatitis
  - Liver transplantation is very rarely indicated if liver failure.

Cholestatic Jaundice

- Common causes:
  - Intrahepatic: Primary biliary cirrhosis, primary sclerosing cholangitis, alcohol, drugs, hepatic infiltration (lymphoma, granuloma, amyloid, metastases), cystic fibrosis, severe bacterial infections, pregnancy, benign recurrent intrahepatic cholestasis, chronic right heart failure
  - Extrahepatic: Carcinoma (ampullary, pancreatic, cholangio-carcinoma), liver metastases, choledocholithiasis, parasitic infection, traumatic biliary strictures, chronic pancreatitis
- Diagnosis:
  - Cholestasis: pruritus, fatigue, dark urine, pale stools, mala-bsorption (vitamins A, D, E and K), weight loss, steatorrhea, osteomalacia, bleeding tendency, xanthelasma
  - Cholangitis: Fever, rigors, pain
  - Underlying condition: Abdominal pain, stricture, irregular hepatomegaly, palpable gallbladder, abdominal mass, occult blood in stool
  - Cholestatic jaundice is characterized by greater elevation of ALP and GGT than aminotransferases; Ultrasonography can distinguish mechanical obstruction and dilatation of biliary tree

- Treatment:
  - Treatment for pruritus: Cholestyramine, rifampicin, naloxone, ondansetron, S-adenosyl methionine, propofol, ursodeoxycholic acid, phenobarbitone, bright light therapy (10000 lux), surgical bypass of the terminal 15% of ileum, plasmapheresis; intractable itching may be an indication for liver transplantation
  - Dietary neutral fat restricted, calorie intake with medium-chain triglycerides (coconut oil), high protein diet, nutritional supplements
  - Vitamin A, D, E and K; oral or parenteral replacement
  - Biliary decompression: Choice between non-surgical and surgical treatment depend upon the cause of obstruction and the clinical state of the patient
  - Common duct stones are treated by endoscopic sphinctero-tomy and removal
  - Inoperable malignant obstruction, a stent is inserted to drain by endoscopy or by the percutaneous route. A laparotomy for by pass with hepaticojejunostomy and Roux-en-Y is the alternative.

Hepatitis A

- Ribonucleic acid (RNA) virus of picornavirus family of enterovirus, is highly infectious
- Spreads by feco-oral route through contamination of water
- Has receptors on hepatocytes and mainly infects liver
- Virus is infectious 2–3 weeks before onset of symptoms during incubation period
- Infectivity persists for 2–3 more weeks during disease progression
- Infection is most common in children, but adult can be infected (30%)
- Source: Water contamination, poor sanitation, overcrowding, selfish (vehicle of transmission)
- Clinical features: Nausea, vomiting, malaise, arthalgia, headache, fever, abdominal pain, anorexia, jaundice (mild/moderate), enlarged, tender liver
- Diagnosis: Raised ALT (200–2000 U/L), raised serum bilirubin, anti-HAV IgM positive (diagnostic)
- Complications: Acute hepatic failure, cholestatic hepatitis, relapsing hepatitis, nephrotic syndrome
- Treatment: Rest till ALT normalizes, antiemetic (if vomiting persists), IV saline (for rehydration, if needed)

- Prevention: Pure drinking water, improvement of sanitation, vaccination of day care staff and nurses specially in intensive care units, close contacts of patients and elderly with other major disease
- Killed vaccine available—single dose or a second dose can be given 6-12 months apart.

CHAPTER 37

Hepatitis E

- Ribonucleic acid (RNA) virus of hepaviridae family of enterovirus
- Endemic in India and Africa
- Spread by contamination of sewerage water
- Adults mostly affected, children affected in 30%
- Only immunocompromised (e.g. liver transplant recipients) may be chronically infected
- Outbreaks occur in monsoon by contamination of water with sewerage over flood
- Clinical features: Prodrome (nausea, vomiting, anorexia, dis-test to taking food), fever (mild), weakness, malaise, jaundice, tender hepatomegaly with smooth surface and sharp margin
- Diagnosis: Elevated serum bilirubin, raised serum ALT, anti-HEV IgM positive (diagnostic), RT-PCR for HEV RNA (confirmatory)
- Infection during pregnancy has high mortality due to risk of acute liver failure
- Management: Mainly symptomatic according to need (e.g. antiemetic if vomiting persists, IV saline for rehydration, etc.)
- Prevention: Education, improvement of sanitation, pure drinking water
- Vaccine: A vaccine of HEV capsid protein is available.

CHAPTER 38

Hepatitis B

- Hepatitis B virus (HBV) infection is a major global public health problem
- Two billion people worldwide are infected, among them 400 people are chronically infected
- Hepatitis B virus is a DNA virus of hepadna family, with outer envelope (HBsAg), core antigen (HBcAg), X-protein (HBx) and precore antigen (HBeAg)
- Classified into eight genotypes, A to H based on nucleotide sequence
- HBV is not directly cytopathic. Hepatic injury is due to immune mediated t-cell response
- Loss of HBsAg indicates viral clearance, but re-emergence can occur in immunosuppressed
- Transmission: HBV is transmitted parenterally, percutaneuosly, by sexual contact, perinatally during delivery of a HBV infected mother and from close contact in first 2 years of life, injection drugs abuse, unscreened blood transfusion, heterosexuality, close contact and sharing of tooth brush and razor of HBV infected individuals and abrasion, cut, etc.
- Progression of disease in chronic infection is inversely related to age 90% perinatal, 20–50 toddlers and 1–2% in adults respectively

- Prevention: Education, universal precaution and vaccination
- Vaccine: 2 types; plasma derived from purified infected patients blood and recombinant vaccine by PCR hybridization; 3 doses at 0, 1 and 6 months
- Indications: All newborn, health workers, homosexuals, multiple sexual partners, injection drug abusers, hemodialysis patients, public safety workers, spouse of patients, sexual partner of patients, household members of HBV carrier, etc.
- Diagnosis: HBsAg (a serological test, hallmark of HBV infection, persistence >6 months implies chronic infection); HBeAg (marker of HBV replication and infectivity, seroconversion from HBeAg to anti-HBe associated with decreased HBV DNA load; HBV DNA (PCR) (detected 2–3 weeks before the appearance of HBsAg, serial HBV DNA determines phase of infection); liver biopsy (asses hepatic necroinflammation and extent of fibrosis); ALT (elevation more than upper normal limit is a biochemical marker); ALT/AST ratio (alteration is indicator of liver damage); Alpha feto- protein (marker of liver cancer); Upper GIT endoscopy (for varices and gastropathy screening and banding of varices)
- Extrahepatic manifestations: serum sickness, polyarteritis nodusa, cryoglobinemia, glomerulonephritis, etc.
- Natural history: Depends on HBV replication, HBV genotype, viral variant, age, gender, race, ethnicity, immune response, alcohol, coinfection with other viruses, e.g. HCV, HDV, HIV.
- Clinical outcome:
  - Acute HBV infection is mild and may remain asymptomatic, can persist for few days with mild prodrome, diagnosed by serological tests, i. e. HBsAg, anti-HBc AgM, resolution of acute HBV signified by loss of HBsAg and detection of anti-HBs

- Chronic hepatitis B persists in 4 phases
  - Immune tolerant phase: HBeAg positive, high HBV DNA, normal ALT; rate of progression of cirrhosis is very low before 40 years age
  - Immune clearance: HBeAg positive, high HBV DNA, Persistent or intermittent elevation of ALT; higher rate of cirrhosis or HCC
  - Inactive carrier phase : HBeAg negative, anti-HBe present, low ALT, low or undetected HBV DNA
  - Reactivation phase: HBeAg negative, anti-HBe positive, high DNA, elevated ALT
- Treatment:
  - Pegylated interferon alpha 2a (HBsAg negative in 28% of patient after 48 weeks of therapy)
  - Nucleos(t)ides analogues:
    - Adefovir 10 mg tablet daily, previously widely used, slow acting antiviral drug, resistance rate very high
    - Lamivudine 100 mg tablet daily, prolonged use leads to resistance
    - Entecavir (0.5 mg), Tenofovir (100 mg), Telbivudine (600 mg) newer drugs suitable for long time use, resistance rate <15%
  - In chronic HBeAg-positive hepatitis B, treatment for 1 year after HBeAg-seroconversion and HBV DNA undetectable on 3 occasions at 6 month apart
  - In chronic HBeAg negative hepatitis B, treatment for 1 year after HBV DNA undetectable on 3 occasions at 6 month apart
  - In HBV cirrhotics treatment is lifelong.

CHAPTER 39

Hepatitis D

- Defective RNA virus, requires HBV for replication
- Mode and routes of transmission same as HBV
- Coinfects simultaneously with HBV or can infect after hepatitis B virus exposure as superinfection
- Coinfection gives rise to acute hepatitis, which is very severe, but can subside with treatment of HBV
- Superinfection with HBV lead to cirrhosis early
- Diagnosis: HDV Ag (Delta antigen) appears in blood early; anti-HDV IgM appears after a short interval; HDV Ag and anti-HDV IgM are diagnostic; HDV RNA (PCR) (specific)
- Management: Pegylated interferon alpha-2a.

Hepatitis C

- Ribonucleic acid (RNA) virus of *flavivirus* family causing chronic liver disease, cirrhosis and hepatocellular carcinoma
- Acute hepatitis is very mild and patients remain asymptomatic for many years
- Chronic liver disease is usually the first manifestation
- Epidemiology: >150 million people are infected worldwide, >2% of people in Asia and Africa
- Hepatitis C transmission occurs through injection drug use, needle stick injury in healthcare settings, heterosexuality, skin piercing (e.g. tattoo), vertical transmission and unscreened blood products, etc.
- There are 6 genotype 1 to 6
- Clinical findings: <15% develop acute hepatitis, upto 80% develop chronic hepatitis, cirrhosis develops 15–20 years after infection, 4% develop hepatocellular carcinoma (HCC)
- Disease progresses rapidly in coinfection with HBV, alcohol, nonalcoholic steatohepatitis
- Extrahepatic manifestations: Cryoglobulinemia, glomerulonephritis, neuropathy, lichen planus, thyroiditis, porphyria, etc.
- Diagnosis: Anti-HCV confirm exposure to HCV; HCV RNA (PCR); AST/ALT usually 1.5–2.5 times more than normal; liver biopsy (assess

hepatic necroinflammation and extent of fibrosis); Fibroscan (assess hepatic fibrosis); USG (hepatic parenchymal echotexture coarse or nodular in cirrhosis)

- Management:
  - Oral drugs: Sofosbuvir, ribavirin, simeprevir, ledipasvir, daclatasvir.
  - Injectable drugs: Pegylated interferon alpha-2a/2b.

CHAPTER 41

Acute Liver Failure

- Clinical syndrome of liver dysfunction, coagulopathy and encephalopathy developing within 26 weeks of onset of symptoms in patients without pre-existing liver disease
- Viral hepatitis is the most common cause worldwide
- Survival depends on the underlying etiology, early treatment and the diligent care of complications
- Complications: Cerebral edema, intracranial hypertension
- Diagnosis: CT (Cerebral edema/intracranial hypertension, rule out other causes of decreased mental status)
- Treatment:

  Grade 1/2 encephalopathy
  - Listing for transplantation
  - Avoid stimulation, avoid sedation if possible
  - Antibiotics: Prophylaxis possibly helpful for unexplained deterioration
  - Lactulose

  Grade 3/4 encephalopathy
  - Tracheal intubation
  - Elevation of head-end of bed
  - Placement of intracranial pressure (ICP) monitoring device

- Immediate treatment of seizures: Mannitol (0.25–1 g/kg IV bolus), hypertonic saline 30% 5–10 mL/h, hyperventilation, barbiturate coma (pentobarbital 3–5 mg/kg IV bolus then 1–3 mg/kg/h or thiopental 5–10 mg/kg IV bolus then 3–5 mg/kg/h)
- Continuous renal replacement.

Infection

- Aseptic techniques
- Antifungal coverage for patients not responding to broad spectrum antibiotics
- Antibiotic prophylaxis possibly helpful but not proven.

Coagulopathy

- Vitamin K: 10 mg IV or subcutaneously
- Fresh frozen plasma (FFP): Only for performing invasive procedures or when active bleeding
- Platelets: If platelet count $<10,000/mm^3$ or for performing invasive procedures
- Recombinant activated factor VII: 40 µg/kg bolus, 30 minutes before procedure if coagulopathy refractory to FFP
- Cryoprecipitate: If fibrinogen <100 mg/dL and active bleeding
- Exchange plasmapheresis: Allows transfusion of large amount of FFP
- PPI or H2 blocker: Prophylaxis for stress ulceration.

CHAPTER 42

Liver Cirrhosis

- May be asymptomatic, but some may have lethargy, fatigability, loss of taste, itching (compensated cirrhosis) or ascites, altered consciousness, hematemesis and melena, epistaxis (decompensated cirrhosis)
- Loss of libido (male), irregular menses and amenorrhea (female)
- History pointing to etiology—surgery, IV drug users, blood transfusion, alcohol intake, family history of liver disease and liver cancer, diabetes mellitus (DM), drugs (e.g. methotrexate, amiodarone)
- Stigmata of chronic liver disease—spider telangiectasia, palmar erythema, Dupuytren's contracture, gynecomastia, testicular atrophy, breast atrophy (female), bruises, purpura, jaundice, splenomegaly, fetor hepaticus, flapping tremor, etc.
- Liver function test (LFT)—normal or altered
- Chronic liver disease screen: Viral markers (HBsAg, Anti-HCV), liver autoantibodies (antinuclear factor, smooth muscle antibody, antimitochondrial antibody), immunoglobulins, ferritin, alpha 1 antitrypsin, serum ceruloplasmin.
- Ultrasonography to see liver echotexture
- Esophagogastroduodenoscopy to detect evidence of portal hypertension.

- Treatment:
  - Treatment of underlying cause, i.e. antiviral for HBV, HCV, D-penicillamine for Wilson's disease, etc.
- Maintenance of nutrition
- Treatment of complications, i.e. beta blocker for portal hypertension, diuretics for ascites
- Liver transplantation in case of decompensated cirrhosis.

Ascites

- Accumulation of excess free fluid in peritoneal cavity
- On examination, bulging flanks, shifting dullness or fluid thrill
- Patients with cirrhosis may exhibit stigmata of chronic liver disease
- Ultrasonography is the best means for confirmation
- Paracentesis may point to the underlying cause
- For classifying serum-ascites albumin gradient (SAAG) is the most useful parameter
- SAAG >1.1g/dL is consistent with ascites secondary to portal hypertension with 98% accuracy
- SAAG <1.1g/dL can occur in ascites due to infection (especially tuberculosis), malignancy or inflammation
- Ascitic fluid neutrophil count >250/mm^3 suggests SBP
- Treatment:
  - Sodium restriction: No added salt in diet, avoid sodium containing and retaining drugs
  - Water restriction is necessary if plasma sodium <125 mmol/L
  - Diuretics: Spironolactone (100–400 mg/day) is the drug of choice. Some also require loop diuretics (furosemide upto 160 mg/day)
  - For refractory ascites: Large volume paracentesis with IV albumin, TIPS, peritoneovenous shunt
  - Treatment of the underlying cause.

CHAPTER 44

Hepatic Encephalopathy

- Syndrome of altered mental status ranging from confusion to coma, secondary to liver cell failure in conjunction with portal systemic shunting
- Precipitating factors: GI bleeding, sepsis, azotemia, sedative or analgesic use, non compliance with medications
- On examination evidences of cirrhosis (spider angioma, palmer erythema, ascites), fetor hepaticus, flapping tremor (asterixis), inability to perform simple mental arithmetics, inability to draw objects (constructional apraxia), hyper-reflexia, bilateral extensor planter responses
- Electroencephalography: Decreased mean cycle frequency; usually not necessary
- Treatment:
  - Identification and treatment of precipitating factors
  - Lactulose: 15–30 mL, 4 times daily, needs to be titrated so that patients experiencing 2–3 loose bowel motions per day
  - Rifaximin: 550 mg twice daily or 400 mg 3 times daily
  - Chronic or refractory case: Liver transplantation.

CHAPTER 45

Portal Hypertension and Esophageal Varices

Essentials of diagnosis:

- Patient of cirrhosis of liver known or unknown
- History of hematemesis and/or melena, hepatic encephalopathy
- Splenomegaly is a cardinal finding. Collateral vessels on anterior abdominal wall (direction of flow is away from umbilicus), caput medusa may be present
- Fetor hepaticus, ascites
- Esophageal varices, gastric varices on esophagogastroduodenoscopy.

Management:

- Management of acute variceal bleeding
- Primary prevention of variceal bleeding:
  - Nonselective beta-blocker, Propranolol (80–160 mg/day) or nadolol at doses that reduce heart rate by 25% from baseline but not below 55–60 beats/min.
- Secondary prevention of variceal bleeding: Endoscopic variceal ligation (EVL)
- Recommendations on use of beta-blocker:
  - Small varices that have not bled:
    - Beta-blocker if there is increased risk of bleeding (Child B/C, red wales on varices).

- In absence of the risk, beta blocker is not recommended. EGD should be repeated in two years.

– Medium/large varices that have not bled:
  - If increased risk of bleeding—Beta-blocker or endoscopic variceal ligation (EVL)
  - In absence of the risks—Beta-blocker is preferred. EVL if there is contraindication or intolerance or non-compliance to beta-blockers.

CHAPTER 46

Variceal Hemorrhage

- Vomiting of fresh blood or clot in a patient with known or suspected cirrhosis of liver
- Passage of black tarry stool or melena may follow
- It is a medical emergency; diagnosis and management should run parallel
- Better to manage it in intensive care unit (ICU) setting
- Treatment:

  Initial measures
  - First step is to assess airway and obtain peripheral venous access with wide bore needle
  - Quick assessment of circulatory status and stigmata of CLD is looked for
  - Basic investigations such as full blood count (FBC), liver function test (LFT), urea and electrolytes are sent and cross matching of blood done
  - Prompt blood volume resuscitation with caution, goal is to maintain hemodynamic stability and Hb of 8 gm/dL
  - Vigorous resuscitation with saline solution should be avoided
  - Oxygen inhalation if patient is in shock
  - Transfusion of fresh frozen plasma (FFP) and platelets are considered in significant coagulopathy and/or thrombocytopenia.

- Vitamin K1 intravenously is routine
- Prophylactic antibiotics: IV ceftriaxone 1 gm/day for 5–7 days
- Frequent monitoring of vital parameters.

Specific measures

- Vasoactive drug should be started in patients with known or suspected cirrhosis of liver; choices are:
    - Vasopressin: Continuous IV infusion of 0.2–0.4 units/min, can be increased to maximum 0.8 units/min. IV nitroglycerine should always be given with it at a dose of 40 mcg/min to a maximum of 400 mcg/min to maintain SBP >90 mm Hg
    - Somatostatin: 250 mcg IV bolus followed by infusion of 250 mcg/hour
    - Octreotide: 50 mcg IV bolus followed by 25–50 mcg/hour
    - Terlipressin: 2 mg IV 6 hourly for 48 hours, can be titrated down to 1 mg 6 hourly.

- Esophagogastroduodenoscopy (EGD) should be performed within 12 hours to make the diagnosis. Endoscopic variceal ligation (EVL) is done if variceal source of hemorrhage is confirmed.

Rescue therapies

- If bleeding can't be controlled or recurs early despite above measures, shunt surgery or TIPS performed
- Balloon tamponade can be used as a temporary measure.

Hepatocellular Carcinoma

- Fifth most common cancer in the world
- Cirrhosis is the most important additional risk factor for hepatocellular carcinoma (HCC)
- Right upper quadrant pain (moderate to severe), dull aching and constant
- Paraneoplastic syndrome includes hypoglycemia, hypercalcemia, thrombocytosis and hypercoagulability with venous thrombosis
- Ultrasonography and alpha-fetoprotein are the surveillance tests for HCC every 6 months
- Diagnosis of HCC include radiology, biopsy and AFP serology
- For lesions >2 cm, typical radiological finding are highly specific; no biopsy is necessary
- Treatment:
  - The Barcelona Clinic Liver Cancer (BCLC) scheme for staging of liver cancer and the treatment strategies that are recommended for each stage
  - Treatment of early HCC has high cure rate
  - Therapeutic techniques include liver resection, liver transplantation, hepatic artery ligation, hepatic artery embolization, chemoembolization, internal radiotherapy, external beam radiotherapy, local ablation with heat, cold, corrosive substances such as ethanol, acetic acid or hot

saline and more recently targeted agents such as raf-kinase or vascular endothelial growth factor (VEGF) inhibitors

- Liver transplantation is the best treatment option for suitable patients with hepatocellular carcinoma.

Secondaries in Liver

- Presentation:
  - Asymtomatic—incidentally detected during abdominal imaging
  - Pain abdomen, lump in abdomen, anorexia, weight loss
  - Symptoms of the primary tumor
  - Hormonal symptoms as in functional neuroendocrine tumors
  - Detected during staging of the primary tumor
- Causes:
  - Colorectal cancers
  - Carcinoma lung
  - Carcinoma stomach
  - Carcinoma pancreas
  - Carcinoma breast
  - Biliary malignancy
  - Malignant neuroendocrine tumors
  - Malignant ovarian tumors.
- Work-up
- Imaging:
  - Ultrasound abdomen: Usually multiple, bulls eye appearance
  - Dynamic CT: Usually on enhancing in arterial phase, but arterial enhancement may be seen in carcinoids and NET,

thyroid tumors, renal cell carcinoma. Portal vein thrombosis unusual
  - FDG PET: To localize tumor else where and to monitor therapeutic response.
- Tumor markers:
  - Carcinoembryonic antigen (CEA), cancer antigen 19.9, cancer antigen 125, chromogranin A (CgA).
- Tissue diagnosis:
  - Best done from the primary site
  - May be done from liver metastasis when primary site is unknown
  - Fine-needle aspiration cytology (FNAC) or liver biopsy may be done
  - Immunohistochemistry and cytokeratin staining may be helpful to ascertain the origin of tumor and to see hormone responsiveness in certain cases.
- Treatment
- Surgery with curative intents
  - In colorectal mets <4 in number in suitable candidate
  - In neuroendocrine tumors (NET) with simple forms of metastasis
  - Liver transplant in diffuse NET metastasis with protracted hormonal symptoms
- Palliative treatment:
  - Chemotherapy
  - Local ablation
  - Transarterial chemoembolization.

CHAPTER 49

Hepatic Hemangioma

- Most prevalent focal mass lesion in the liver, 5–10% in general population
- Large or multiple lesions associated with pain, mass effect, congestive heart failure or consumption coagulopathy
- Vascular bruit may be heard
- Lesions may enlarge in pregnancy and with oral contraceptive pill (OCP)
- Risk of hemorrhagic complication in pregnancy is low
- Imaging techniques confirm the diagnosis without biopsy
- Treatment: Arterial embolization (bleeding adenomas); surgical excision (>5 cm, adenomas in men).

Hepatic Adenoma

- Women > men, usually within child-bearing age
- Patients may present with right upper quadrant mass
- Hepatic tenderness is associated with rupture
- Serum biochemical tests may be normal
- Risk of malignant transformation in men 40–50%
- Usually solitary (70–80)
- Risk factors: Exposure to OCP, anabolic steroid or danazol
- Treatment: Arterial embolization (bleeding adenomas); surgical excision (>5 cm, adenomas in men).

CHAPTER 51

Portal Vein Thrombosis

- Formation of thrombus in portal vein, either extrahepatic or intrahepatic portion or both
- Causes:
  - Umbilical sepsis and omphalitis
  - Umbilical vein cannulation
  - Abdominal sepsis or surgery
  - Abdominal trauma
  - Inflammatory condition of abdomen: Pancreatitis, diverticulitis, portal pyemia
  - Procoagulant states—occult or overt myeloproliferative disorders, paroxysmal nocturnal hemoglobinuria, factor V Leiden, prothrombin gene mutation, Protein C, S and antithrombin III deficiency, pregnancy
  - Liver cirrhosis
  - Hepatocellular carcinoma—tumor thrombosis.
- Natural history, etiology and management of extrahepatic portal vein obstruction (EHPVO) is different from portal vein thrombosis occurring in setting of liver cirrhosis and hepatocellular carcinoma
- In East, umbilical sepsis and intra-abdominal sepsis leading to portal vein thrombosis in extrahepatic portion during childhood is the most frequent type. While in the west, presentation in adulthood in background of procoagulant condition is more frequent.

- Clinical features:
  - Acute/recent thrombosis: Pain abdomen, fever, mild ascites, bloody stools with mesenteric ischemia
  - Chronic thrombosis: Asymptomatic, Recurrent gastroesophageal bleeding, hypersplenism, ascites is usually transient secondary to bleeding or surgery. Portal biliopathy may present with obstructive jaundice and cholangitis. Hepatocellular failure is usually absent and occurs late in course of disease.
- Diagnosis:
  - Ultrasound examination with Doppler study
  - Contrast enhanced computed tomography (CECT) abdomen or CT splenoportogram or magnetic resonance venogram
  - Screening for factor V leiden, protein C and S activity, Antithrombin III level, JAK 2 mutation studies.
- Management:
  - In acute presentation or recent thrombosis anticoagulation can establish patency of portal vein and prevent cavernoma formation
  - No role of anticoagulation in chronic thrombosis with cavernoma formation
  - Anticoagulation should be considered in acute to subacute thrombosis even in setting of liver cirrhosis
  - In partial thrombosis > 50% of lumen and/superior mesenteric vein extension anticoagulation may be considered.
  - Anticoagulation should be continued till at least 3 months. If recurrent thrombosis occurs or underlying procoagulant state persist, lifelong therapy may be needed

- Gastroesophageal varices should be ligated and obliterated before starting anticoagulation
- Beta-blocker may be used for primary prophylaxis if anticoagulation is not considered
- Splenectomy and shunt surgery is rarely required in refractory cases.

CHAPTER 52

Budd-Chiari Syndrome

- Characterized by hepatic outflow obstruction
- Causes are clotting disorders, cancer, coinfection, congenital web and cryptogenic
- Presentation ranging from asymptomatic to fulminant hepatic failure
- Ascites, upper abdominal pain, hepatomegaly, hepatic encephalopathy are common, often upper gastrointestinal bleeding
- Serum bilirubin usually not over 2 mg/dL, raised alkaline phosphatase, reduced serum albumin, increased transaminase and prothrombin time, hyponatremia due to protein-losing enteropathy
- Ascitic fluid analysis reveals exudative and high serum albumin ascetic albumin gradient (SAAG)
- Heart failure and constrictive pericarditis should be excluded carefully
- Ultrasonography, Doppler study, CT scan and MRI gives supportive evidence
- Liver biopsy shows zone 3 sinusoidal distension and pooling, also excludes cirrhosis of liver
- Hepatic venography and inferior vena cavography are diagnostic; describes the level of obstruction

- Treatment:
  - Elimination or treatment of the cause
  - Management of ascites, portal hypertension
  - Surgical—portocaval shunt, transjugular intrahepatic portosystemic shunts (TIPS), liver transplantation.

Drug-induced Liver Injury

Type of liver injury	***Commonly responsible drugs***
Acute hepatocellular injury	Isoniazid rifampicin, methyldopa, keto-conazole, diclofenac
Fulminant hepatitis	Paracetamol
Cholestatic hepatitis	Chloropromazine, erythromycin, amoxicillin—clavulanate, clarithromycin
Chronic hepatitis	Methotrexate, lisinopril
Autoimmune hepatitis	Nitrofuratoin, minocycline
Steatohepatitis	Amiodarone, griseofulvin
Cirrhosis	Methotrexate, amiodarone
Adenoma	Anabolic steroid, contraceptive pill
Cholangiocarcinoma	Thorotrast, vinyl chloride, arsenic

- Management: Immediate discontinuation of offending drug; in most but not all cases liver injury subsides
- When injury continues as autoimmune hepatitis and recovery fails even with discontinuation of offending drug, corticosteroid treatment is commonly used

- Cholestyramine may benefit pruritus
- Methotrexate causes liver cirrhosis in high doses over long period of time; severe fibrosis and cirrhosis are relatively common (17%); liver biopsy should be done after every 1–1.5 gm cumulative dose.

Nonalcoholic Fatty Liver Disease

- Nonalcoholic fatty liver disease (NAFLD) is defined as macrovesicular fat accumulation in >5% of hepatocytes
- NAFLD is considered as the hepatic manifestation of metabolic syndrome, characterized the presence of 3 or more of the following:
  - Abdominal obesity (waist circumference >102 cm in men, >88 cm in women)
  - Hypertriglyceridemia (>150 mg/dL)
  - Low HDL levels (<40 mg/dL in men, <50 mg/dL in women)
  - Hypertension (>130/80 mm/Hg) and
  - High fasting glucose levels (>110 mg/dL).
- Asymptomatic, persistent fatigue, malaise or upper abdominal discomfort
- Steatohepatitis (NASH) may progress to cirrhosis and present with ascites, jaundice, encephalopathy and liver failure
- Comorbidities include cardiovascular disease (CVD), diabetes, obstructive sleep apnea (OSA), colonic adenomas, hyperuricemia, pancreatic steatosis, hypothyroidism and polycystic ovary syndrome (PCOS)
- Raised AST or ALT level may be the only abnormality with NAFLD and AST-to-ALT ratio of less than 1 may occur in NASH

- Liver is hyperechogenic or bright in USG
- Loss of intensity on T1-weighted images in MRI may be useful in identifying focal fat
- Liver biopsy is the gold standard for diagnosing NAFLD and NASH
- Treatment:
  - Dietary advice: Weight loss (7%–10%), moderate caloric restriction (aim to reduce daily calories by 500–700 kcal), reduce saturated fatty acids and high fructose from diet, omega-3 fatty acid replacement, regular coffee consumption (2–3 cups/day)
  - Moderate exercise, maximum 4–5 times weekly for 30–45 minutes each time
  - Pharmacotherapy: Vitamin E (800–1000 IU daily), pioglitazone 30–45 mg daily, pentoxifylline, statins
  - Bariatric surgery: Roux-en-Y gastric bypass (RYGB), Laparoscopic adjustable gastric banding (LAGB), sleeve gastrectomy.

Alcoholic Liver Disease

- Spectrum comprising of simple steatosis, alcoholic hepatitis and cirrhosis
- The risk increases with daily intake of >30 gm/day The risk of developing cirrhosis increases with >60–80 gm/day for men for 10 or more years and >30 gm/day for women. Only 35% of heavy drinkers develop alcoholic liver disease (ALD)
- Factors like sex, obesity, drinking pattern, dietary factor, non-sex linked genetic factors and cigarette smoking are involved in development of advanced ALD
- Alcoholic steatosis:
  - Simple alcoholic steatosis may be asymptomatic. Diagnosis may be done following USG screening.
- Alcoholic hepatitis:
  - Alcoholic hepatitis may present as alcohol dependence syndrome with anxiety, tremor, sweating, abdominal pain. Mild form may be asymptomatic with raised enzymes. AST>ALT.
  - Severe form of hepatitis presents with fever, jaundice, ascites, encephalopathy, leukocytosis, hepatorenal syndrome
  - Physical finding show features of chronic liver disease. Jaundice, ascites, spider naevi, hepatic bruit, edema, encephalopathy. Features like parotid gland enlargement, Dupuytren contractures and malnourishment are also noted.

- Investigation:
  - Ultrasonography: Fatty hepatomegaly to cirrhotic changes
  - Liver function test (LFT) deranged with AST>ALT, raised bilirubin, raised gamma-glutamyl transpeptidase (GGT) coagulopathy, leukocytosis, impaired renal function
  - Endoscopy: Varices may be seen.
- Alcoholic cirrhosis in compensated state may be asymptomatic. In decompensated state features of CLD like ascites, edema, jaundice, variceal bleed, hepatorenal syndrome, hepatic encephalopathy are present
- Treatment:
  - In mild form of ALD, alcohol abstinence with improved nutrition is the mainstay of treatment as some are malnourished. Vitamin supplementation is warranted
  - Severe form of alcoholic hepatitis may require ICU care. Treatment options include steroids, pentoxifylline for those with discriminant function >32. Others include anti-TNF therapy, antioxidants like silymarin, S-adenosylmethionine, antifibrotic (colchicine).
  - Liver transplantation.
- Prognostic scoring system: Maddrey discriminant function (DF), MELD score, Lille score, Glasgow alcoholic hepatitis score.

Autoimmune Hepatitis

- Fatigue, jaundice, upper abdominal discomfort, mild pruritus, myalgia, diarrhea, fever, Cushingoid features or none at presentation
- Physical findings: Hepatomegaly, jaundice, splenomegaly, ascites, encephalopathy, concurrent immune disease or none
- Laboratory findings: Elevated AST, hypergammaglobulinemia, increased IgG, hyperbilirubinemia, raised ALP ≥2 fold upper normal limit
- Immunoserologic markers: Smooth muscle antibody (SMA), antinuclear antibody (ANA), antibody to liver-kidney microsome type 1 (anti-LKM1), antisoluble liver antigen, perinuclear anti-neutrophil cytoplasmic antibody (pANCA)
- Indications for treatment:

  Absolute indications
  - Clinical: Incapacitating symptoms, relentless clinical progression
  - Laboratory: AST ≥10-fold ULN or AST ≥5-fold ULN and gamma-globulin ≥2-fold ULN
  - Histologic: Bridging necrosis, multilobular necrosis

Relative indications

- Clinical: Mild or no symptoms
- Laboratory: AST 3- to 9.9-fold ULN or AST ≥5-fold ULN and gamma globulin <2-fold ULN
- Histologic: Interface hepatitis.

None indications

- Clinical: Asymptomatic with minimal laboratory changes, previous intolerance of prednisone and/or azathioprine
- Laboratory: AST <3-fold ULN, severe cytopenia
- Histologic: Inactive cirrhosis, portal hepatitis, decompensated cirrhosis with variceal bleeding.

- Treatment:

  Initial regimens for treating autoimmune hepatitis

  - High dose monotherapy: Prednisolone (Week 1: 60 mg, week 2: 40 mg, week 3:30 mg, week 4: 30 mg); early maintenance until end-point agreed with patient 20 mg.

  Initial monotherapy with subsequent azathioprine

  - Week 1: Prednisolone 20–30 mg, week 2: prednisolone 20–30 mg, week 3: prednisolone 20–30 mg, week: prednisolone 20–30 mg and Azathioprine 1–2 mg/kg if responding and bilirubin <100 μmol/L; early maintenance until end-point agreed with patient; tapering dose to 5–10 mg by 1 year.

  Combination therapy from outset

  - Week 1: Prednisolone 30 mg and azathioprine 50 mg, week 2: Prednisolone 20 mg and azathioprine 50 mg, week 3: Prednisolone 15 mg and azathioprine 50 mg; early maintenance until end-point agreed with patient prednisolone 10 mg and azathioprine 50 mg.

Primary Biliary Cirrhosis

- Strong female to male predominance, 9:1
- Usually female of 40–60 years are affected
- Pruritus is the most common initial complaint, worse on the limbs; fatigue is also common; jaundice is prominent late in the disease; hematemesis, melena may develop
- Skin xanthomas, hepatomegaly and splenomegaly may be found on physical examination
- Associated autoimmune diseases such as sicca syndrome, systemic sclerosis, rheumatoid arthritis may be present
- Diagnosis of primary biliary cirrhosis (PBC) is established when two of following three criteria are met:
  - Biochemical evidence of cholestasis: Raised ALP
  - Presence of antimitochondrial antibody (AMA)
  - Histologic evidence of nonsuppurative destructive cholangitis and destruction of interlobular bile ducts.
- Treatment:
  - The only recommended drug for PBC is ursodeoxycholic acid (UDCA), dose: 13–15 mg/kg/day in two divided doses; if bile acid sequestrants are required, 2–4 hour before or after food intake

- To relieve pruritus, options are: Cholestyramine (bile acid sequestrants) 4–16 g/day orally' rifampicin 300 mg/day, naltrexone (an opioid antagonist) 50 mg/day
- Treatment of complications: Osteopenia/Osteoporosis: calcium 1000–1500 mg and vitamin D 1000 IU in diet and as supplements, alendronate 70 mg orally weekly in absence of acid reflux or varices; portal hypertension: beta-blocker, endoscopic variceal ligation (EVL)
- Liver transplantation remains the only effective treatment for those with end-stage disease
- Screening family members by alkaline phosphate (ALP).

Primary Sclerosing Cholangitis

- Occurs mainly in young men, male: female ratio 2:1, age 25–40 years
- Typical symptoms are right upper quadrant abdominal discomfort, fatigue, pruritus, weight loss; fever with chills are uncommon; many are asymptomatic
- Physical examination may reveal jaundice, hepatomegaly, splenomegaly
- 60–80% patients with PSC have concomitant IBD, most often ulcerative colitis
- Cholangiocarcinoma may develop in 10–30% patients
- Liver function test (LFT) shows cholestatic pattern, bilirubin usually normal
- Cholangiography (MRCP or ERCP) is the key investigation; shows characteristic multifocal strictures and segmental dilatations of biliary tree
- Treatment:
  - Role of ursodeoxycholic acid (UDCA) is doubtful
  - Corticosteroid, azathioprine, methotrexate and cyclosparine may be beneficial
  - Management of complications:
    - Acute cholangitis: Broad-spectrum antibiotics

  - Extrahepatic bile duct obstruction: "Dominant stricture" on cholangiography—stent or balloon dilatation at ERCP
  - Metabolic bone disease: Calcium and Vitamin-D supplement.
- Full colonoscopy with biopsies with a new diagnosis of PSC with no past history or symptoms of IBD; survillence colonoscopy with biopsies in concomitant PSC and IBD
- Liver transplantation: Indicated in young patients with PSC and in advanced liver disease.

Hemochromatosis

- Classically refers to *HFE*-mediated genetic iron overload
- Excess iron deposition leads to end organ damage, typically involves the liver first and may also involve pancreas, heart, pituitary gland and others
- Mostly asymptomatic at diagnosis and identified by laboratory screening or family history
- Diagnosis is typically made earlier in men, while women are protected by menstruation
- Symptomatic patients often present with unexplained fatigue, arthralgia, weight loss, abdominal pain and reduced libido
- In advanced cases: Hepatomegaly, raised liver enzymes, cirrhosis, diabetes mellitus, heart failure, dysarrhythmia, leaden grey skin pigmentation
- Current diagnostic markers include: Iron studies, liver biopsy, gene analysis and response to therapy
- Combination threshold of transferin saturation >50% with ferritin >300 mcg/L for men and transferin saturation >45% with ferritin >200 mcg/L for women are suggestive
- Liver biopsy: To confirm diagnosis and staging; also allows determination of hepatic iron index (HII). HII >1.9 is highly suggestive

- Genetic testing identify common mutations
- Treatment:
  - Weekly phlebotomy of 500 mL blood (250 mg iron) until serum ferritin <50 mcg/L
  - Maintainance phlebotomy: 2–4 times a year to maintain serum ferritin 50–100 mcg/L
  - Avoid alcohol and vitamin C, which increase iron absorption
  - First degree relatives should be screened and if confirmed phlebotomy should be started even if asymptomatic.

CHAPTER 60

Wilson's Disease

- Wilson's disease is an inherited disorder of copper homeostasis
- It is caused by mutations in the gene *ATP7B*
- Clinical features: Chronic hepatitis, cirrhosis, fulminant liver failure usually in adolescents and young adults
- Neurologic manifestations: Behavioral changes, decreased performance status, spasticity and rigidity, ataxia, dystonia and tremors
- Diagnosis: Serum ceruloplasmin decreased by 50% of lower normal value, increased urinary excretion of copper (>100 µgm/24 h), Kayser-Fleischer (KF) rings in the cornea by slit lamp examination, elevated hepatic copper level (>250 µgm copper/g dry liver), genetic testing may be useful in screening families
- Treatment:
  - Early diagnosis is essential and treatment should be lifelong
  - Avoid copper containing foods (shellfish, liver, nuts, mushrooms and chocolate)
  - D-penicillamine (chelates copper and increases urinary excretion)

    Adults

    - Start with incremental doses, 125–250 mg/day increased by 250 mg increments every 4–7 days to a maximum

of 1000–1500 mg/day in 2–4 divided doses taken 1h before meal; maintenance dose 750–1500 mg/day in 2–3 divided doses
  - Pyridoxine 25–50 mg/day.

Children
  - Start with 20 mg/kg/day, increased to 250 mg in 2–3 divided doses
- Trientine (chelator promotes urinary copper excretion)
  - Indication: Who cannot tolerate D-penicillamine
  - Usual dose:750–1500 mg/day in 2–3 divided doses, taken 1 hour before or 3 hour after meals
  - Maintenance therapy: 750 or 1000 mg/day
- Zinc
  - Indication: Maintenance therapy in patients stabilized with D-penicillamine or trientine
  - First line therapy in asymptomatic and pre-symptomatic patients
  - Usual dose: 150 mg elemental zinc/day (for children <50 kg body weight) in 3 divided doses, 30 minutes before meal
- Acute hemolysis in Wilson's disease: Exchange transfusion
- Pregnancy in women with Wilson's disease:
  - Pregnancy is safe
  - Continued treatment with D-penicillamine, trientine or zinc has been well-tolerated by mothers
  - Prolonged interruption of treatment may potentiate risk of hepatic insufficiency
  - First two trimesters: 750-1000 mg/day of either D-penicillamine or trientine in well-controlled patients
  - Last trimester: Dose reduction to 500 mg/day.
- Breastfeeding under chelation therapy is not recommended.

Amebic Liver Abscess

- Amebiasis affects in 10% world population
- Pregnancy, malnutrition, alcoholism, glucocorticoid use, malignancy are contributory factors
- Caused by *Entamoeba histolytica*. It has two form—tropozoite and cyst
- Trophozoites exist only in the host
- Cysts survive outside the host in water, soil and food
- Amebic liver abscess common in man, rare in children
- Latent period may be many years
- Clinical features: Pain, intermittent fever, night sweats, nausea, vomiting, weight loss, jaundice (indicates poor prognosis), enlarged, tender liver, friction rub, etc.
- Diagnosis: USG (shows space occupying lesion with filling defect containing fluid); CT (more specific); serology (hemagglutination test); aspiration, reddish-brown pus (anchovy sauce pus)
- Complications: Intraperitoneal, intrathoracic and pericardial rupture (fatal), multiorgan failure
- Treatment: Metronidazole —750 mg three times daily by mouth or IV for 7–10 days; Tinidazole or chloroquine may be substituted for metronidazole
- Treatment response usually occurs within 96 hours.

Pyogenic Liver Abscess

- Abscess secondary to biliary disease (29–69%), cryptogenic (40%)
- Causes: Gallbladder empyema, perforated peptic ulcer disease, subphrenic abscess, appendicitis, diverticulitis, Crohn's disease, etc.
- Causative organisms: *Escherichia coli, Klebsiela pneumonie, Pseudomonas aeruginosa, Proteus species, Haemophilus, Legionella, Staphylococcus, Enterococcus*, Beta-hemolytic *Streptococcus*
- Clinical features: Fever, chills, rigor, anorexia, nausea, vomiting, malaise, weakness, diarrhea, cough, chest pain, tender hepatomegaly, right upper quadrant pain, jaundice (rare), etc.
- Diagnosis: Anemia, leukocytosis, raised ESR; elevated ALP; blood culture positive (50%); USG (fluid-filled lesion), CT (diagnoses as small as 1 cm lesion); abscess drainage and pus culture (confirmatory)
- Treatment: Appropriate antibiotic for 6 weeks, 2 weeks followed by oral administration and treatment of underlying cause.

Hydatid Disease

- Hydatid disease is due to larval or cyst stage of infection by the tapeworm, *Echinococcus granulosus*, which lives in dogs. Humans, sheep and cattle are intermediate hosts
- Hydatid cyst in the liver may have no symptoms or low-grade fever, pain, tender hepatomegaly, dyspnea and hemoptysis (when cysts ruptures into lungs), anaphylactic reaction, cholangitis, pyogenic liver abscesses, pancreatitis, portal hypertension or Budd-Chiari syndrome
- Enzyme-linked immunosorbent assay (ELISA) is the best serologic assay for diagnosis
- Plain abdominal radiographs may show ring-like calcifications; ultrasonography and CT confirm the diagnosis with intracystic septations and daughter cyst formation; presence of protoscolices or acid-fast hooklets in the cyst fluid confirms the diagnosis
- Treatment:
  - Medical treatment: Albendazole 10–15 mg/kg/day in 1 month courses separated by 14 days intervals (3–6 courses)
  - Percutaneous-Aspiration injection-reaspiration (PAIR) of scodicidal agent and of hydatid cyst

Indications

- Nonechoic lesion ≥5 cm
- Cysts with daughter cysts
- Multiple cysts if accessible to puncture
- Patients who fail to respond to medical therapy alone
- Patients in whom surgery is contraindicated
- Patient who refuse surgery
- Patients who relapse after surgery.

– Surgery:

  Indications

  - Large cysts with multiple daughter cysts
  - Cysts that may rupture (spontaneously or as a result of trauma)
  - Cysts communicating with biliary tree and/or exerting pressure on adjacent vital organs
  - Cysts in the lung, brain, kidney, bones and other organs.

– 4 days of treatment with albendazole before PAIR or surgery is mandatory and should continue for 1 month after the procedure.

Leptospirosis

- One of the most common zoonoses having wide range of animal reservoir
- Acquired by contaminated urine, soil or water
- Anicteric leptospirosis presents with flue-like illness, conjunctival suffusion followed by abdominal cramps, tenderness, hepatomegaly, rarely aseptic meningitis
- Weil's syndrome presents with deep jaundice, renal failure and hemorrhagic manifestations
- Elevated ALT, serum bilirubin, creatine kinase, neutrophilic leukocytosis and thrombocytopenia
- Positive blood culture, urine culture and positive MAT; detection of DNA by PCR is diagnostic
- Treatment:
  - Bed rest; complicated case and Weil's syndrome need ICU care
  - Supportive treatment for jaundice, hemorrhagic manifestations (blood transfusion, FFP, platelet concentrate)
  - Careful monitoring of renal function, early detection of abnormality and prompt management
  - Doxycycline 100 mg bd for one week or IV penicillin 900 mg qid for one week or IV ceftriaxone 1 gm daily for one week.

Familial Hyperbilirubinemia

Gilbert's Syndrome

- Inherited as autosomal dominant trait caused by mutation of uridine diphosphate glucuronyltransferase enzyme
- Defined as benign, familial, mild, unconjugated hyperbilirubinemia (serum bilirubin 17–85 μmol/L)
- Raised serum bilirubin is not due to hemolysis
- Routine liver function tests are normal
- Hepatic histology shows no change
- Affects 2–5% of the population
- Patients with Gilbert's syndrome have deficiency in hepatic bilirubin glucuronidation
- Clinical features: Jaundice mild and intermittent; aggravated by intercurrent infection or fasting; may be associated with malaise, nausea and often discomfort over the liver
- Symptoms are probably no greater than in normal controls
- There is no physical signs; spleen is not palpable
- Diagnostic tests include increase in serum bilirubin on fasting, that falls on taking phenobarbitone, which induces the hepatic conjugating enzyme

- Patients with Gilbert's syndrome have a normal life expectancy and reassurance is the only necessary treatment.

Crigler-Najjar Syndrome

- This form of familial nonhemolytic jaundice is associated with very high serum unconjugated bilirubin
- Inheritance is autosomal recessive
- Deficiency of conjugating enzyme can be demonstrated in the liver

  Type I
  - In affected patients, serum bilirubin is >350 μmol/L
  - No bilirubin conjugating enzyme can be detected in liver
  - Bile contains no bilirubin conjugate
  - Since, serum bilirubin eventually stabilizes, the patient must have some alternative pathway of bilirubin metabolism
  - Phototherapy gives temporary benefit
  - Phototherapy degrades unconjugated bilirubin into products including lumi bilirubin, which is water soluble and can be secreted into the bile.

  Type II
  - This form of familial nonhemolytic jaundice has an autosomal dominant inheritance
  - Bilirubin conjugating enzyme in the liver is reduced to <10% normal
  - Serum bilirubin usually does not exceed 350 μmol/L
  - Jaundice is present in about half of the patients within the first year of life, but can occur as late as 30 years of age
  - Acute exacerbations of hyperbilirubinemia may occur during fasting or intercurrent illnesses and bilirubin encephalopathy can develop

- Jaundice responds to phenobarbitone and patients survive into adulthood.
- The distinction between type I and type II Crigler-Najjar syndrome is made by observing the response to phenobarbitone
- There is no response in patients with type I and type II is confirmed if serum bilirubin falls by more than 25%
- An alternative approach is to analyse duodenal bile after phenobarbitone; in type II there is increase in biliary mono- and diconjugates.

Dubin-Johnson Syndrome

- A chronic, benign, intermittent jaundice with conjugated hyperbilirubinemia and bilirubinuria
- Autosomal recessive and is most frequent in the Middle East among Iranian Jews
- There is reduced canalicular excretion of organic anions, including bilirubin
- The defect in canalicular transporter gene explains the diagnostic pattern seen in the prolonged BSP test; after intravenous injection of BSP there is an initial fall in serum level, but the value at 120 minutes exceeds that seen at 45 minutes due to regurgitation into the circulation of its glutathione conjugate, which is normally excreted into bile via MRP-2
- The liver, macroscopically is greenish-black (black-liver jaundice)
- Sections the liver cells show brown pigment, which is neither iron not bile
- Though, it is a chronic disease, the course is mild and no treatment is necessary.

Rotor Syndrome

- Resembles Dubin-Johnson syndrome in being a form of chronic familial conjugated hyperbilirubinemia
- Main difference is absence of brown pigment in hepatocytes in Rotor syndrome
- Electron microscopy may shows abnormalities of mitochondria and peroxisomes.

CHAPTER 66

Intrahepatic Cholestasis of Pregnancy

- Relatively benign illness occurs in 2nd or 3rd trimester of gestation
- Usual presentation is itching followed by jaundice; nausea, vomiting and abdominal pain may associate; excoriations are common
- Half of the patients of intrahepatic cholestasis of pregnancy (ICP) have history of similar illness following use of oral contraceptive pills
- Symptoms usually progress till delivery and disappear dramatically within 48 hours after delivery
- Biochemical abnormalities: Increased serum bilirubin, alkaline phosphatase, gamma GT and mildly increased SGPT/SGOT; become normal within few weeks
- Long-term follow-up reveals increased incidence of gallstone and other gallbladder diseases
- Treatment:
  - Nutritional support
  - Injection Vitamin K (phytonadione) 10 mg IV daily for 3 days; one dose at least 6 hrs before delivery
  - Dexamethasone 12 mg/day for 7 days; then tapered over 3 days

- Ursodeoxycholic acid (UDCA) 1 gm/day upto 2 gm/day
- Phenobarbitone,S-adenosyl-L-methionine and choles-tyramine may be alternate options
- Delivery is the end point of sufferings, but ICP frequently reappears in subsequent pregnancies.

CHAPTER 67

Acute Fatty Liver of Pregnancy

- Potentially fatal but rare; occurs during pregnancy between 34–36 weeks
- Nausea, vomiting, abdominal pain followed by jaundice is the common presentation
- In severe cases encephalopathy, renal failure, hemorrhage, disseminated intravascular coagulation (DIC), sometimes ascites may develop
- Signs of preeclampsia found in 50% cases
- Differential diagnosis: Acute viral hepatitis, drug-induced hepatitis, toxemia of pregnancy
- Serum ammonia and amino acid level, blood urea, serum creatinine elevated. Serum bilirubin (mostly conjugated) and SGPT raised (rarely above 500 IU/mL), prothrombin time prolonged, but gamma globulin is normal
- Hypoglycemia is profound, sometimes hyponatremia and hyperkalemia are seen
- Ultrasonography of liver shows diffuse increased echogenicity; low attenuation at CT scan
- Treatment:
  - Mild to moderate cases should be managed at high care unit, severe cases at ICU

- Careful observation, supportive management for hemorrhage, coagulopathy, renal failure, electrolytes derangement and other complications
- Proton pump inhibitor can be given to prevent esophagitis and hemorrhage
- Pregnancy should be delivered in severe cases
- Careful observation for the postpartum complications
- Hepatic transplantation is rarely necessary.

HELLP Syndrome

- Syndrome comprises ***H**emolysis, **E**levated **L**iver enzymes and **L**ow **P**latelet count*
- Occurs usually in 3rd trimester and postpartum periods; life-threatening for both mother and fetus
- Maternal mortality is high in severe cases (Platelet <50,000/cmm)
- Presents with hypertension, proteinuria, nausea, vomiting, pain abdomen, headache, edema
- Serum glutamic pyruvic transaminase SGPT usually >500 IU/L, Serum bilirubin usually <5 mg/dL
- Coagulopathy, hypoglycemia, renal failure, later on hepatic encephalopathy may complicate the situation and leads to maternal and fetal mortality
- Imaging: Hepatic rupture or infarction can be detected (rare)
- Liver biopsy: Patchy or extensive necrosis with hemorrhage can be found (rarely done)
- Treatment:
  - Preferred management at ICU
  - Management of complications; correction of renal failure
  - Platelet transfusion is recommended if thrombocytopenia <20,000/cmm

- Prompt delivery if >34 weeks of gestation; if <34 weeks, both fetus and mother stable, corticosteroid should be given for fetal lung maturity
- Recurrence is common in subsequent pregnancies.

CHAPTER 69

Benign Recurrent Intrahepatic Cholestasis

- Rare disease of recurrent episodes of cholestatic jaundice
- Onset with itching, occasionally with influenza-type illness, vomiting and abdominal pain (25–50%). There is often fatigue, anorexia and weight loss
- Serum alkaline phosphatase levels increase, but transaminases are virtually normal. Jaundice appears and typically persists for 3–4 months
- Hepatic histology shows cholestasis with bile plugs, portal zone expansion, mononuclear cells and some liver cell degeneration, mainly in zone 1. Hepatic histology and liver function are normal on remission
- Etiology: Autosomal recessive; gene locus mapped to the *FIC1* locus as for *PFIC1*
- Treatment: Attacks are self-limiting and vary in duration; corticosteroid probably of little benefit. 30 mg daily for 6 weeks may be given in severe cases; ursodeoxycholic acid is controversial, but may reduce bilirubin and ALT, dose 300 mg daily orally12 hourly; rifampicin has been highly effective in some cases at 600 mg daily orally.

CHAPTER 70

Liver Transplantation

Mayo Clinic Definition of Liver Transplantation

A liver transplant is a surgical procedure to remove a diseased liver and replace it with a healthy liver from a donor. Most liver transplant operations use livers from deceased donors, though a liver may also come from a living donor.

Indications for Liver Transplantation

- Chronic hepatitis C, chronic hepatitis B, autoimmune hepatitis, alcoholic liver disease, primary biliary cirrhosis, primary sclerosing cholangitis, metabolic liver disease (e.g. inborn errors of metabolism), hepatocellular carcinoma, fulminant hepatic failure
- Cirrhotic patients should be referred for transplantation when there is evidence of hepatic dysfunction [Child-Turcotte-Pugh (CTP) >7 and Model of End-stage liver disease (MELD) >10] or when they experience their first major complication (ascites, variceal bleeding, or hepatic encephalopathy)
- Biliary atresia is a common indication for liver transplantation in pediatric patients.

Contraindications to Liver Transplantation

- Absolute
- Psychological, physical and social inability to tolerate the procedure, active sepsis, metastatic malignancy (except hepatic neuroendocrine tumors), cholangiocarcinoma (except trial protocols with neoadjuvant therapy and staging laparotomy), AIDS, advanced cardiopulmonary disease
- Relative (higher risk)
- Age more than 65 or less than 2 years, prior-portacaval shunt, prior complex hepatobiliary surgery, portal vein thrombosis, retransplant, multiorgan transplants, morbid obesity, HIV, serum creatine more than 1.7 mg/dL (150 μ mol/L), chronic renal failure (requires combined liver/kidney transplantation).

Transplant Listing Criteria

Status 1A and 1B patients have first priority for receiving cadaveric liver grafts. These patients and those with MELD score >25 are recertified every 7 days.

- Status 1A 18 years or older with:
  - Fulminant hepatic failure (onset encephalopathy <8 weeks of jaundice)
    - *and* ventricular dependence, renal support and INR >2.0
    - *or* acute decompensation due to Wilson's disease
  - Primary non-function or hepatic artery thrombosis (HAT)* within ≤7 days or liver graft implantation
    - *and* aspartate transaminase >3000 U/L and either INR >2.5, or acidosis
    - *or* anhepatic following graft removal

* If HAT ≤14 days not meeting above criteria are listed with the highest MELD score of 40.

- Status 1B age less than 18 years:
  - Chronic liver disease requiring ICU care with one of the following:
    - Ventilator dependence
    - Gastrointestinal bleeding with >30 mL/kg red cells ≤24 hour
    - Renal support
    - Glasgow coma score <10 within previous 48 hour
  - *and* calculated model for end-stage liver disease (MELD) or pediatric end-stage liver disease (PELD) >25 points
- All others †
- Based on increasing MELD/PELD scores.

† Hepatocellular carcinoma — a single lesion 2 cm diameter or more is given extra points Regional Review Boards review exceptions to MELD.

Drugs used in Post-transplant Immunosuppression

Cyclosporine, tacrolimus, sirolimus, azathioprine, everolimus, mycophenolate, corticosteroids.

Complications following transplantation

Acute graft rejection, vascular thrombosis, biliary leak or stricture, infection, malignancy, adverse effects of immunosuppressant drugs.

Laboratory studies to assess evidence of rejection and drug effects

Complete blood count; electrolytes; blood urea nitrogen and creatinine; liver function tests; cultures of blood, urine or sputum; cyclosporine or tacrolimus level; chest radiography; abdominal ultrasonography, CT scan or ERCP as indicated.

Consultations

- Early admission should be arranged for any infection other than minor infections. Transplant physicians should be involved early in the course for evaluation and management, if rejection is suspected.

CHAPTER 71

Acute Cholecystitis

- Ninety five percent associated with obstruction of the gallbladder neck or cystic duct by a gallstone
- About 5–10% acute cholecystitis in adults occur in the absence of stone, usually associated with critical condition like major nonbilliary surgery, multiple injuries, etc.
- Sufferers are often obese, female, over 40, but no type, age or sex is immune
- Pain occurs at late night or early morning, usually in the right upper abdomen or epigastrium, referred to the angle of the right scapula or right shoulder and rarely to the left, lasts for 30–60 minutes without relief, attacks precipitated by heavy meal or fatty food and in severe cases, patient may present with fever
- Physical finding: Patients appear ill, temperature rises, jaundice indicates associated stone in the gallbladder, Murphy sign positive
- Investigations: Leukocyte count raised, in febrile patients blood culture may be positive; USG is the first choice with 96% accuracy; cholescintigraphy is second line option; serum amylase should be measured to detect acute pancreatitis
- Treatment: NPO, intravenous fluid; For pain NSAID (in moderate pain), pethidine (in severe pain); antibiotics (second or third

generation cephalosporin or combination of quinolone with metronidazole); in patient with features of sepsis piperacilin plus tazobactam with an aminoglycoside can be used

- Surgery: Early cholecystectomy (within 1 week) is superior to delayed cholecystectomy (2 to 3 months later); urgent surgery can be done when cholecystitis progress in spite of optimal medical therapy and when complications develop (e.g. empyema or perforation).

Chronic Cholecystitis

- Commonest gallbladder disease
- Almost always associated with stone
- Recurrent attacks of upper abdominal pain
- Abdominal distention or epigastric discomfort especially after meal temporarily relieved by belching
- Physical finding: Local tenderness over the gallbladder; positive Murphy sign highly suggestive
- Investigations: Gallstone within a fibrosed gallbladder with thickened wall on USG; esophagogastroduodenoscopy (EGD) to rule out the gastric or duodenal ulcer
- Treatment: Low fat diet, weight reduction, symptomatic patients advised to undergo elective laparoscopic cholecystectomy.

CHAPTER 73

Cholelithiasis

- Gallstone cholelithiasis formation is multifactorial; genetics, lifestyle, obesity, dietary factors, age, sex, cirrhosis, diabetes mellitus, hereditary spherocytosis or sickle cell disease may have impact on stone formation
- Cholesterol (51–95%) is the predominant component of stone; other contents are calcium carbonate, phosphate, bicarbonate and pulmitate, phosphorus, glycoprotein and mucopolysaccharides
- The major type of gallstone are: cholesterol stone, black pigment stone and brown pigment stone
- Usually asymptomatic and diagnosed incidentally by imaging
- Around 8–10% with asymptomatic gallstone develop symptoms within 5 years and only 5% require surgery
- Treatment: Prophylactic cholesystectomy for asymptomatic gallstone should not be performed, elective cholecystectomy is the best treatment for symptomatic patients
- Patients who are unfit or refuse surgery can be managed by nonsurgical treatment
- Ursodeoxycholic acid (UDCA) 10 mg/kg/day for at least two years may be effective

- Criteria for UDCA response: Patient must be compliant, symptoms mild to moderate, cystic duct patent, radiolucent stone, preferably floating, <15 mm in diameter, stone attenuation value <100 Hansfield unit
- Overall success rate for drug therapy are 40–60%
- Extracorporeal shock wave therapy can be given for fragmentation.

Choledocholithiasis

- Stone in the bile duct causes intermittent obstruction of bile duct
- Usually asymptomatic. Sometimes presented with biliary pain, cholangitis and pancreatitis
- Physical examination reveals normal. May present with jaundice and pain
- Jaundice without pain favors malignancy rather than stone
- Raised alkaline phosphatase and serum bilirubin (<10 mg/dL) is the common laboratory finding. Transient raise in serum glutamate-pyruvate transaminase (SGPT) indicate passage of stone
- Ultrasonography, endoscopic ultrasound (EUS), magnetic resonance cholangiopancreatography (MRCP), endoscopic retrograde cholangiopancreatography (ERCP) and percutaneous, tetrahydrocannabinol (THC) can be used as diagnostic tool
- Endoscopic stone removal during ERCP followed by laparoscopic cholecystectomy is the treatment of choice nowaday. Lesser stone crash using spyglass cholangioscope during ERCP introduced by some advance endoscopy centers.

Postcholecystectomy Syndrome

Definition

Postcholecystectomy syndrome consists of abdominal symptoms of biliary and non biliary disorder that takes place after cholecystectomy.

Prevelance

5–40% suffer after cholecystectomy.

Symptoms

- Dyspepsia
- Flatulence
- Bloating
- Right upper abdominal pain/discomfort (may be mild persistent to severe episodic)
- Vomiting.

Pathophysiology and Etiology

- Reservior function of gallbladder is lost leading to altered bile flow and enterohepatic circulation
- Bile reflux—gastritis, esophagitis
- Missed gallbladder stones in common bite duct (CBD)
- Stones primarily formed in CBD
- Cystic duct remnant—neuroma

- Fixed narrowing from the inflammation and fibrosis with asymptomatic passage of stone
- Sphincter Oddi dysfunction and ampulla spasm.

Investigation

- Complete blood count (CBC) to exclude infection
- Liver function test (LFT) (ALT, AST, Bilirubin, ALP, GGT, PT)
- Lipase
- Hepatitis panel
- Electrocardiography (ECG)
- Chest X-ray to exclude diaphragmatic diseases
- Esophagogastroduodenoscopy (EGD)
- Endoscopic ultrasound (EUS)
- MRCP, ERCP and SOM (Sphincter Oddi manometry).

Differential Diagnosis

- Extraintestinal disorder—ischemic heart disease (IHD)
- Nonbiliary gastrointestinal disorder—peplic ulcer disease (PUD)
- Biliary disorder—choledocholithiasis
- Irritable bowel syndrome (IBS)
- Psychiatric disease.

Treatment

Treatment according to cause. Avoidance of fatty food, frequent small meals.

Drugs

- Antispasmodic:
  - Hyoscyamine butylbromide
  - High dose calcium channel blocker
  - Nitrates.

Endoscopic Intervention

- ERCP sphincterotomy when SOD with significant hypertonia of sphincter (biliary/pancreatic)
- Remnant cystic duct stone removal.

Sphincter of Oddi Dysfunction

Definition

Sphincter of Oddi dysfunction (SOD) is the cause of pancreaticobiliary type abdominal pain due to increased tonicity of pancreatic and biliary sphincter.

- Common in middle aged female.

Prevalence

10–20% in postcholecystectomy patient.

Pathogenesis

- Stenosis due to fibrosis and/or inflammation
- Dyskinesia of sphincteric smooth muscles leads to intermittent obstruction due to spasm.

Clinical Features

- Episodic pain lasts more than 30 minute once a year. More common in postcholecystectomy or in patient with gallbladder stone
- But may be present without gallstone disease.
  - Persistent or recurrent abdominal pain (biliary type) post-cholecystectomy
  - Recurrent pancreatitis

- Recurrent biliary type pain with intact gallbladder and without cholelithiasis.

Classification

Modified Milwaukee System

Type 1
- Biliary type pain
- ALT/AST/ALP—1.1 × ULN
- Bile duct dilatation >9 mm

Type 2 Pain + one II of and III

Type 3 Only pain.

Differential Diagnosis

- Gastroesophageal reflux disease (GERD)
- Fatty liver
- Irritable bowel syndrome (IBS)
- Biliary microlithiasis.

Diagnosis

Noninvasive

- Liver function test (LFT)
- Lipase
- Ultrasonography (plain + post fatty food)
- Hepatobiliary iminodiacetic acid (HIDA) scan
- Secretion/CCK stimulated USG, MRCP, EUS

Invasive

- ERCP with SOM (normal—30 mmHg) (3-fold risk of post ERCP pancreatitis).

Treatment

Low fat diet to avoid stimulation of pancreaticobiliary stimulation.

Drugs

Medical therapy should be tried in all patient with III and less severe type II before sphincterotomy

- Nifedipine, nitrates
- Octreotide
- Antispasmodics—hyoscyamine
- Low dose tricyclic.

Some physicians try cholecystectomy before ERCP.

Endoscopic Intervention

- Empirical sphincterotomy in type I and type II, abnormal SOM required for type III
- Post sphincterotomy temporary cannulation with pancreatic stent reduces the complication rate.

Choledochal Cyst

- Congenital disease characterized by cystic dilatation of one or more segments of the biliary tree
- Though, it is a childhood disease, but may present in adult life; female predominance (4:1)
- Choledochal cysts are classified as follows:
  - Type-I: Cystic, segmental fusiform dilatation of the extrahepatic bile duct
  - Type-II: Cyst forming diverticulum
  - Type-III: Cystic dilatation of the distal column of the bile duct
  - Type-IV: Type 1 anomaly along with intrahepatic bile duct
- Type I and IV are most common
- Infantile form present with prolonged cholestatic; if not diagnosed earlier, can lead to biliary cirrhosis and portal hypertension
- In adult patients, there is jaundice, abdominal pain and abdominal lump
- Jaundice is intermittent and cholestatic type associated with fever
- Complication are recurrent cholangitis, portal vein thrombosis, liver abscess, carcinoma
- USG and CT scan detect the cyst, but MRCP is the first choice for detecting cyst

- Treatment:
  - Cholangitis can be managed with antibiotics
  - Radical excision of cyst with hepaticoduodenectomy with Roux-en-Y anastomosis is the treatment of choice to reduce the subsequent risk of adenocarcinoma
  - For type–III cyst—endoscopic sphincterotomy or unroofing of the cyst
  - For extensive disease, hepatectomy or liver transplantation.

Carcinoma Gallbladder

- Gallbladder (GB) cancer is most typically diagnosed in the seventh decade of life, with a median age of 62–66 years
- Risk of GB cancer raises with cholesterol gallstones, primary sclerosing cholangitis, ulcerative colitis, liver flukes, chronic *Salmonella typhi*, paratyphi infections, *Helicobacter* infection, organochlorine pesticide (OCP), methyldopa, pesticides, obesity, anomalous pancreaticobiliary duct junction, choledochal cysts, gallbladder polyps, calcified (porcelain) gallbladder
- Pain in the right upper quadrant, fever, nausea, vomiting, bloating, weight loss, jaundice, palpable mass in the right upper quadrant (Courvoisier sign), periumbilical lymphadenopathy (Sister Mary Joseph nodules), left supraclavicular adenopathy (Virchow node)
- CBC, LFT (raised ALP and bilirubin), CA 19.9, CEA, USG (mass can be identified in 50–75% cases)
- CT scan of abdomen and chest, MRCP, EUS, ERCP, FDG-PET, staging laparoscopy
- Treatment:
  Surgery
  - Stage IA disease (T1 N0 M0): Simple cholecystectomy
  - Stage IB (T2 N0 M0): Extended cholecystectomy
  - Stage IIB (T1-3N1 M0): Extended cholecystectomy

- Stage III (T4, any N, M0): Gallbladder cancer is not surgically curable

Radiation therapy

- After curative resections with close or positive microscopic margins, gross macroscopic residual disease, palliative debulking, tumors beyond the mucosa

Chemotherapy

- 5-FU plus concurrent radiation therapy, gemcitabine or fluoropyrimidine, gemcitabine plus cisplatin or gemcitabine plus capecitabine

Palliative therapy

- Endoscopic or percutaneous stent insertion.

• Prognosis: Poor, 5-year survival rates 15–20%
• Advanced gallbladder cancer: 1 year survival rate <5%
• Median survival is 2–4 months.

Cholangiocarcinoma

- Older age
- Deep jaundice followed by pruritus
- Weakness and weight loss
- Liver is large and smooth
- Serum bilirubin, alkaline phosphatase (ALP) and gamma glutamyltransferase (GGT) may be very high
- Raised CA 19.9 (in PSC sensitivity is 50–60%) and CEA
- Ultrasound scan/helical CT/MRI/MRCP/PET scan
- Cytology at ERCP or percutaneous drainage
- Angiography—hepatic artery and portal vein involvement
- Magnetic resonance angiography (MRA) and CT angiography
- New techniques—endoscopic USG, intraductal USG and direct cholangioscopy
- Treatment:

  Surgery
  - Distal cholangiocarcinoma: pancreatoduodenectomy
  - Spread along the common bile duct: Hepatic resection and pancreatoduodenectomy
  - Mid-bile duct cancer: Resected with excision of the biliary tree and hilar lymphadenectomy

- Typical hilar (Klatskin) tumor: Resected by an extended right or left hepatectomy
- Biliary tree is excised and proximal bile duct(s) drained into a Roux-en-Y loop of intestine
- Radical hilar lymphadenectomy
- Local resection can be considered for Bismuth type I and II tumors with low perioperative mortality

Adjuvant chemotherapy or radiotherapy

- No role

Liver transplantation

- In general, cholangiocarcinoma is a contraindication for liver transplantation

Nonsurgical palliation

- Endoprosthesis across the stricture either by the endoscopic or percutaneous route
- Intraduct photodynamic therapy combined with stenting in patients with unresectable cholangiocarcinoma

Surgical palliation

- Anastomosis of jejunum to the segment III duct in left lobe
- If recurrent stent blockage occurs, surgical bypass can be considered.

Periampullary Carcinoma

- Most arise in head of the pancreas, distal bile duct, ampulla of Vater (papilla) and rarely duodenum
- Peaks in sixth and seventh decades of age
- Gradual and progressive jaundice, itching, pain in epigastrium, back or right upper quadrant, weight loss, weakness, steatorrhea and diarrhea
- Physical examination: Jaundice, weight loss, enlarged and palpable gallbladder, hepatomegaly with sharp, smooth and firm edge
- Anemia, raised ESR, serum bilirubin and ALP, prolonged prothombin time, raised C-reactive protein and raised CA 19.9
- Diagnosis and staging by CT, MRI, EUS, ERCP
- Treatment:
  - Resection: Pancreaticoduodenectomy (Whipple's operation)
  - Palliative procedures:
    - Endoscopic biliary stent insertion
    - When the endoscopic approach fails, a percutaneous or combined percutaneous/endoscopic approach can be used
    - Surgical biliary bypass in unresectable patients (gastroenterostomy as well as choledochojejunostomy)

- Duodenal stenting (in gastric outlet and duodenal stenosis)
- Celiac plexus neurolysis (can provide good pain relief)
- Chemical neurolysis
- Palliative chemotherapy—gemcitabine, 5-FU for locally unresectable or metastatic pancreatic carcinoma
- Molecular therapy—erlotinib.

CHAPTER 81

Acute Pancreatitis

- Acute pancreatitis is defined clinically with two of the following criteria: (1) epigastric pain, consistent with the disease, (2) a serum amylase or lipase greater than three times ULN or (3) radiologic imaging consistent with the diagnosis, usually using CT or MRI
- Abdominal pain is dull, boring, steady, sudden in onset, gradually intensifies, radiates directly through abdomen to the back and discomfort frequently improves in the supine position
- Physical findings: Fever, palpitation, hypotension, abdominal tenderness, muscular guarding, distention, jaundice, hematemesis or melena, Cullen sign (bluish discoloration around umbilicus), Grey-Turner sign (reddish-brown discoloration along the flanks)
- Complications: Acute pseudocyst, intra-abdominal infections, pancreatic abscess, intra-abdominal hemorrhage, colon perforation and multiorgan failure
- Severe acute pancreatitis according to Atlanta classification:
  - Evidence of organ failure (SBP below 90 mmHg, PaO_2 60 mm Hg or lower, serum creatinine level 2 mg/dL or lower, gastrointestinal bleeding amounting to 500 mL or more in 24 hours)
  - Local complications (e.g. necrosis, abscess, pseudocyst)
  - Ranson score of 3 or higher or APACHE score of 8 or higher

- Glasgow criteria for prognosis in acute pancreatitis: More than three implies severe disease.
  - Age >55 years
  - PO_2 <8 kPa (60 mm Hg)
  - White blood cell count (WBC) >15 × 10^9/L
  - Albumin <32 g/L
  - Serum calcium <2 mmol/L
  - Glucose >10 mmol/L
  - Urea >16 mmol/L (after rehydration)
  - Alanine aminotransferase (ALT) >200 U/L
  - Lactate dehydrogenase (LDH) >600 U/L
- Laboratory studies:
  - Serum amylase and lipase, liver-associated enzymes, blood urea nitrogen (BUN), creatinine and electrolyte, complete blood count (CBC), hematocrit, C-reactive protein (CRP), arterial blood gas values, serum lactic dehydrogenase (LDH) and bicarbonate, immunoglobulin G4 (IgG4)
  - ALT >150 U/L (suggests gallstone pancreatitis and a more fulminant disease course)
  - WBC count >12,000/μL and hematocrit >47% at admission is a sensitive measure of more severe disease
  - CRP level >150 mg/L within the first 72 hours of disease correlate with the presence of necrosis.
- Ultrasonography, dynamic spiral CT scanning, EUS, MRI and ERCP
- Treatment:
  - NPO
  - Intravenous fluid resuscitation; both crystalloids and colloids is most effective within the first 12–24 hours (this usually involves administration of several liters of fluid as a bolus, followed by continuous infusion at a rate of 250–500 mL/h)

Urine output (>0.5 mL/kg/h) can be followed up as a markers of adequate hydration

- Enteral feeding should be introduced as pain, anorexia resolves and patient regains appetite; diet should be low in fat and protein
- O_2 inhalation
- Analgesics (tramadol, pethidine)
- ICU support (in shock, respiratory failure, renal failure, GI hemorrhage or multiorgan failure)
- Imipenem-cilastatin, cefuroxime reduces the risk of intra-abdominal infection
- Gallstone pancreatitis: Cholecystectomy
- Recurrent idiopathic pancreatitis: Cholecystectomy

Pancreatic duct disruption

- Image-guided percutaneous placement of a drainage tube into the fluid collection; stent or tube placement via ERCP; in refractory cases, distal pancreaticoduodenectomy or a Whipple's procedure

Large or symptomatic pseudocysts

- Percutaneous aspiration, endoscopic transpapillary or transmural techniques or surgical management

Infected pancreatic necrosis

- Image-guided aspiration; necrosectomy

Pancreatic abscess

- Percutaneous catheter drainage and antibiotics; surgical debridement and drainage

• Prevention:
  - Gallstone pancreatitis: Cholecystectomy
  - Idiopathic recurrent pancreatitis: Cholecystectomy
  - Alcohol abstinence.

Chronic Pancreatitis

- Intermittent severe abdominal pain, postprandial exacerbation of pain, diarrhea, steatorrhea and weight loss with decreased subcutaneous fat, temporal wasting and sunken supraclavicular fossa
- Complications: Pseudocysts, pancreatic ascites, obstructive jaundice, portal or splenic vein thrombosis, peptic ulcer, duodenal stenosis
- Ultrasound, CT (atrophy, calcification or ductal dilatation), abdominal X-ray (calcification), Magnetic resonance cholangiopancreatography (MRCP), endoscopic ultrasound
- Tests of pancreatic function: Collection of pure pancreatic juice after secretin injection (gold standard), fecal pancreatic elastase test
- Treatment:
  - Alcohol and tobacco abstinence
  - For pain relief: NSAID, narcotics, non-narcotics (antidepressant, gabapentin/pregabalin), oral pancreatic enzyme supplements (at least 30,000 units of lipase), antioxidants, octreotide, celiac plexus neurolysis
  - Medium-chain triglyceride therapy

- Proton pump inhibitors (PPI)
- Cobalamin and vitamin B12
- Surgical or endoscopic therapy for pancreatic pseudocyst, abscess, fistula, ascites, papillary stenosis, pancreatic duct strictures, gastric outlet obstruction, variceal hemorrhage.

Pancreatic Carcinoma

- Head of the pancreas is the most common site for carcinoma; approximately 90% are adenocarcinoma arising from dactular epithelium, but may also develop from pancreatic acinar cell, lining of the lower bile duct and the ampulla of Vater
- Male and female ratio 2:1 and the peak incidence is in the sixth and seventh decades
- Predisposing factors are genetic (Kras gene mutation), smoking, obesity, alcohol, type 2 diabetes mellitus, chronic pancreatitis
- Pain, weight loss and obstructive jaundice are usually presenting complaints
- Patients are icterus, hepatomegaly, gallbladder may be palpable (in 50% cases), spleen is enlarged (if there is splenic vein thrombosis), Virchow's gland present
- Pancreatic cancer produces prothrombotic tendency that leads to venous thrombosis
- Serum bilirubin and alkaline phosphatase are raised; CA 19.9 has 79% sensitivity and 82% specificity; imaging modalities for diagnosis and staging of pancreatic cancer include ultrasonography, contrast enhanced CT, magnetic resonance imaging (MRI), endoscopic USG and endoscopic retrograde cholangiopancreatography (ERCP).

- Treatment:
  - If resectable, Whipple's operation is the treatment of choice
  - Adjuvant therapy with 5-flurouracil (5-FU)and folinic acid may have some role
  - Palliative procedure for advanced case include endoscopic biliary stent insertion, surgical biliary bypass, bile duct and duodenal stenting, celiac plexus neurolysis and palliative chemotherapy with gemcitabine and 5-FU
  - Erlotinib, an epidermal growth factor receptor inhibitor, is associated with better prognosis
  - Long-term survival is poor; 5 years survival after pancreatico-duodenectomy is 10–20%.

Index

D

G

H

I

J

P

R

S

T

U